Collaborative Practice in Primary and Community Care

T0186689

The effective delivery of primary care requires the good working of a multi-professional team who provide that care. This accessible and concise text explores the ways in which primary care teams can collaborate well to advance the quality of clinical care and enhance collaborative working across the healthcare system as a whole.

Taking a workbook approach, and including examples, narratives, case histories and further reading, *Collaborative Practice in Primary and Community Care* brings together theory and good practice to offer the reader viable models for achieving excellence. Addressing specific challenges to practising collaboratively throughout, it contains chapters exploring the contemporary context of primary care, collaboration with patients, collaboration between different professional groups, collaboration amongst organisations, and the respective roles of education and technology in promoting collaboration.

Written by a multi-professional selection of experienced authors, practitioners and educators, this textbook is designed for a wide audience of healthcare professionals with an interest in primary care.

Sanjiv Ahluwalia is Postgraduate Dean, Heath Education England (North Central and East London), UK.

John Spicer is Head of Primary Care Education and Development, Health Education England (South London), UK.

Karen Storey is National Primary Care Lead Nurse, NHS England and Improvement, UK.

CAIPE Collaborative Practice Series

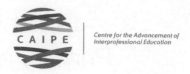

CAIPE | Centre for the Advancement of Interprofessional Education

The *CAIPE Collaborative Practice Series* is an essential forum for sharing research and practice in interprofessional education. Drawing on the expertise of its editorial board, the series focusses on improving collaborative practice and, in that way, improving the quality of care and people's experiences of it.

Written by experienced teachers, practitioners and researchers from across the health and social care professions, the books in the series are:

- designed for professionals and students interested in working more collaboratively
- focused on areas of practice where interprofessional collaboration is an urgent priority
- sourced from across a wide range of practice settings, including child and family practice, public health and critical care
- concise, accessible and readable

CAIPE (Centre for the Advancement of Interprofessional Education) is an independent think tank. It aims to promote and develop interprofessional education with and through its individual, corporate and student members, in collaboration with like-minded organisations in the UK and overseas, for the benefit of patients and clients.

Founded in 1987, CAIPE is a charity and company limited by guarantee which promotes and develops interprofessional education with and through its members. It works with like-minded organisations in the UK and overseas to improve collaborative practice, patient safety and quality of care by professions learning and working together. CAIPE's contributions to IPE include publications, development workshops, consultancy, commissioned studies and international partnerships, projects and networks.

CAIPE not only offers expertise and experience, but also provides an independent perspective which can facilitate collaboration across the boundaries between education and health, health and social care, and beyond. Membership of CAIPE is open to individuals, students and organisations such as academic institutions, independent and public service providers in the UK and overseas. For further information about CAIPE and other benefits of membership go to www.caipe.org.uk

Series Editors: Hugh Barr and Marion Helme
Maggie Hutchings, Bournemouth University, UK and Alison Machin, Northumbria University, UK

Published Titles

Collaborative Practice in Critical Care Settings
A Workbook
Scott Reeves, Janet Alexanian, Deborah Kendall-Gallagher, Todd Dorman, Simon Kitto

For more information about this series, please visit: www.routledge.com/CAIPE-Collaborative-Practice-Series/book-series/CAIPE

Collaborative Practice in Primary and Community Care

Edited by
Sanjiv Ahluwalia,
John Spicer
and Karen Storey

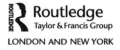

Routledge
Taylor & Francis Group

LONDON AND NEW YORK

First published 2020
by Routledge
2 Park Square, Milton Park, Abingdon, Oxon OX14 4RN

and by Routledge
52 Vanderbilt Avenue, New York, NY 10017

Routledge is an imprint of the Taylor & Francis Group, an informa business

British Library Cataloguing-in-Publication Data
A catalogue record for this book is available from the British Library

Library of Congress Cataloging-in-Publication Data
A catalog record for this book has been requested

ISBN: 978-1-138-59275-9 (hbk)
ISBN: 978-1-138-59278-0 (pbk)
ISBN: 978-0-429-48980-8 (ebk)

Typeset in Sabon
by Apex CoVantage, LLC

Contents

Contributors

Sanjiv Ahluwalia is Postgraduate Dean for Health Education England's North Central East London Team. He has broad experience in clinical education and its management, most recently focussing on the strategic development of multi-professional education at Health Education England while continuing to work as a general medical practitioner. He is completing a doctorate at the Institute of Education, University of London.

Eleni Chambers has worked in health and social care for thirty years, in both service delivery and research settings. She is a long-term user of health and social care services and is passionate about involvement, her interest originating from activism in service delivery settings. She works freelance for a variety of organisations, is a trustee for the National Survivor User Network (NSUN), a Public Representative of Sheffield Clinical Commissioning Group's (CCG's) Strategic Patient Engagement, Experience and Equality Committee and a member of the INVOLVE National Advisory Group (NIHR). She has a particular interest in involving communities who are marginalised and/or not usually involved and is currently doing a PhD in involvement in palliative care research.

Ruth Chambers OBE has worked as a general practitioner (GP) for more than thirty-five years in different practices alongside many lead roles in academia, Royal College of General Practitioners (RCGP), Department of Health (DoH) and learning and development, with various clinical interests – all focussed on disseminating best practices in the clinical management of long-term conditions (LTCs) and patient care. She is the clinical chair of Stoke-on-Trent CCG and clinical lead for technology enabled care services (TECS) for the Staffordshire STP's digital work stream. She is an honorary professor at Staffordshire and Keele Universities.

Katie Coleman works part time as a GP partner at The City Road Medical Centre, a busy inner-city training practice, which she established in 1999 in collaboration with Dr Jo Sauvage. She is the Islington CCG governing board GP lead for patient and public participation and the chief clinical information officer, leading on the development of integrated care records for Islington residents in collaboration with other CCGs across North London Partners in health and social care. In addition she is the North London Partners clinical lead in primary care and care closer to home, providing strategic direction on the development of care closer to home integration networks and quality improvement support teams (QISTs), access to GP services and social prescribing. Katie has recently taken up a GP director role for the Islington GP federation. Katie.coleman@nhs.net; @k8coleman24

Ann Griffin is a doctor of medicine and a doctor of education. She has an academic post as a clinical professor in medical education research at UCL Medical School, London. Ann is the deputy director of the school, director for the Research Department of Medical Education (RDME) and head of Department for Research and is lead for postgraduate programmes and scholarship and sub dean for quality. She works clinically in general practice in North London and is an honorary consultant North Central London. Her research interests include methodological innovations in medical education research, medical regulation, educational quality, professional identity, interprofessional education and transitions in medical education and training. www.ucl.ac.uk/slms/people/show.php?UPI=AGRIF93: a.griffin@ucl.ac.uk; @DrAnnGriffin

Graeme Jeffs has worked as a social worker and family therapist and in a range of roles across the health and social care for the last twenty years. He has in the past been a professional adviser to the Department for Education on children's mental health policy and currently works within the National Health Service (NHS) introducing digital transformation to primary care in England.

Elizabeth Mills is Associate Professor in Clinical Pharmacy and Pharmacy Education at UCL School of Pharmacy. She is also Academic and Educational Strategic Lead at Green Light Pharmacy. She started her career working in community pharmacy and is passionate about the contribution that community pharmacy can make to the NHS. She completed a PhD in which she developed and evaluated a competency framework for pharmacists working in primary care. Since completing her PhD, she has spent her career developing education and training to enable community pharmacists to work collaboratively and become truly integrated members of the primary care team. Her research has focussed on educational issues relevant to the pharmacy profession, and she has a national profile in this respect in two key areas: pre-registration training quality assurance and professional development frameworks. @DrLizzieMills

Catherine O'Keeffe is a registered nurse and doctor of education. She holds honorary academic posts with UCL's IoE as a teaching fellow and as a senior lecturer with KCL's Faculty of Life Science and Medicine. Catherine has extensive experience of strategic clinical educational leadership for postgraduate medical and multiprofessional education in London, nationally and internationally. She has led the development of research and publications in areas including: teaching and learning across the healthcare professionals, faculty development, assessment and appraisal in postgraduate medical education. Catherine works for Health Education England (HEE) and is currently on secondment at GSTT as Associate Director of Education where she is developing the education strategy across the trust.

Stuart Rutland is a paramedic from the South East of England; he first started working for a local ambulance trust in 1996 and for the last ten years has been working in the development of paramedics to better meet the needs of their patients. He has worked in general practice for the last five years, developing the role of the advanced paramedic in primary care. Recently he began a training position in an acute trust as an advanced clinical practitioner in the emergency department whilst continuing to keep strong ties with primary care. He has a long background in education guest lecturing at universities across the South East and London and holds the position of chief examination officer for The College of Paramedics, delivering a biannual competence assessment for paramedics working in primary and urgent care. He has also just completed a secondment as a clinical fellow for Health Education England and last year completed his master's degree at Surrey University. stuart.rutland@nhs.net

Marc Schmid is Director of Redmoor Health and Redmoor Communications CIC, which provide digital training and deployment support for front-line staff and NHS organisations. He has more than twenty years' experience of working in public relations and communications across the NHS and local government. In addition to this he is director at the Newsacademy, which provides media programmes in schools with a focus on educating about health-related issues. In his spare time he is also a junior rugby union coach for Wigan RUFC Under 12s. @marcschmid, @redmoorhealth, www.redmoorhealth.co.uk

Jo Sauvage graduated from University College London Medical School in 1988. She is a part-time GP at the City Road Medical Centre, London. She became a GP in 1997 and committed to working in inner London, establishing her south Islington practice nineteen years ago, with partner Dr Katie Coleman, in a deprived and under-doctored area of central London. She continues to play a significant role as a front-line GP in her local community and continues to be passionate about training future GPs and mentoring clinical colleagues to become future leaders in healthcare. Jo is Chair of Islington CCG, having previously been Vice-Chair (Clinical) since the inception of the CCG. She has many years' experience as a clinical leader working ensuring the transformational changes within the NHS remain clinically led, both within North Central London, the London region and England as a whole, as elected regional representative on the NHS Clinical Commissioners Board. Through the significant span of her roles and responsibilities, she is able to understand the 'end-to-end issues' that affect both patients and staff working across the health and care sector. As such, she is able to illustrate the meaning and importance of collaboration within general practice at all levels and how this will be a vital ingredient in the planning and delivery of good care.

John Spicer is a GP in Croydon, South London, and the head of primary care education for Health Education England [South London]. He maintains interests in clinical law and ethics, which he taught for many years at St George's University of London, interprofessional practice and education, and the medical humanities. He is a trustee of the London Arts and Health Forum. He is committed to, and an advocate of, generalist practice as the best intervention clinicians can make to the health of individuals and populations. Previous publications have included *A Handbook of Primary Care Ethics* (with Andrew Papanikitas), *Primary Care Ethics* (with Deborah Bowman) and *Genetics in Primary Care* (with Imran Rafi). John.Spicer@hee.nhs.uk; @johnspicer3

Karen Storey is the National Primary Care Nursing Lead in NHS England NHS/Improvement leading on the General Practice Nursing Ten Point Plan to support recruitment, retention and return of the nursing workforce in general practice. Prior to this, she was primary care lead nurse (workforce) at Health Education England West Midlands leading on Training Hubs. She has held previous positions as Primary Care Nurse Facilitator in a CCG, and Clinical Lead Nurse for an NHS Walk – In Centre. She has a background as a General Practice Nurse, Nurse Practitioner, Independent Nurse Prescriber and an MSc in Health Studies. Karen has held various national roles to develop the HEE GPN career framework, nurse lead on the HEE primary care workforce commission 'The future of primary care creating teams for tomorrow', HEE national general practice nursing workforce plan 'Recognise, Reform, Rethink'. Karen's role as associate lecturer in the Faculty of Applied Health Care Research University of Birmingham has included visits to primary care in Denmark, Netherlands and China. She has a particular interest in growing nursing leadership in primary care, and has developed a shared leadership programme for primary care known as 'Triumvirate leadership'. Karen is a Queen's Nurse and is a graduate of the QNI Executive Nurse Leaders Programme.

Chris Warwick is a GP in Surrey and Sussex and head of Health Education England (HEE) KSS GP School. His involvement with paramedic advanced practice training dates back to the earliest pilot courses for paramedics to explore their full potential as primary care clinicians. Through his work in a large, multi-professional training practice, to his leadership of the primary care educational network in KSS, Chris has maintained a championing approach to allied professionals' contribution to the primary care workforce of the future. His own research into learning needs in International Medical Graduates has shaped national policy in terms of how overseas recruits are inducted and supported into the complexity of the NHS, and he understands the interrelationships amongst myriad organisations which constitute the modern NHS. Christopher.warwick@hee.nhs.uk; @drchriswarwick

Foreword

General practice has been the bedrock in the care of community health since the inception of the NHS in 1948. Those early days of the NHS General Practice relied then, as they do now, on the skills, expertise, care and compassion of many multi-professional healthcare staff including doctors, nurses, allied health professions and pharmacists. Whilst the scale and approach of general practice has changed radically since those early days, the collaboration of care staff continues to be a great source of support and pride to the nation.

The ethos of patient centredness and holism have been key approaches in managing the complexities of health issues in the community, alongside health promotion and increasing specialisation of treatments and management that have come along with increasing medical advances.

We welcome this new book that celebrates the collaboration in primary and community care that this book is about. We have both seen in our professional work the interprofessional collaboration centred on the needs of the patient, their carers, families and communities. It is vital that we celebrate the professionalism and multiprofessional approaches in primary care that have led to many innovations and health improvements.

As Chief Nursing Officer I am sure that it is important that we continue to develop and support our nurses in general practice to ensure that they can continue to drive change and lead care in general practice. We must recognise the importance of general practice and community nursing as the leader of all nurses in England. As a leader in general practice and healthcare professional education, Professor Gregory has supported team learning and care whilst respecting professional attributes and strengths. Together we have worked locally, regionally and nationally to support high-quality patient care. Such care is best achieved when we all work together, when we feel personally and professionally safe and know that we are supported to work together by our leaders. Together we support the multi-disciplinary team and the crucial import of collaboration.

This book is a welcome addition to the accumulating evidence of collaboration within primary and community care, and between primary and community care and wider system partners including patients and patient groups, secondary care, social care, local government, the third sector and many others. Primary care is the bedrock of our NHS. UK and international evidence demonstrate that sustainable, affordable healthcare systems are built on strong primary care. There is much evidence from the UK, across Europe, including Holland, Scandinavia, Canada, Australasia and latterly reinvigorated by the Affordable Care Act (Obamacare) in the United States of America. There is a considerable body of evidence, not least the seminal work of Barbara Starfield,[1] that strong primary care supports safe, high-quality, patient-centred care. This book further draws upon this evidence and demonstrates that this care is further improved by collaboration.

The NHS Long Term Plan (for England)[2] is an ambitious plan to improve care for patients and the health of citizens for the next ten years. It will soon be supported by the NHS People Plan. This plan is broad with key foci on ensuring the best start in life, world-class care for major health problems and supporting healthy aging. Amongst the methods outlined in the plan for delivery of these ambitions are key promises to increase collaboration in primary and community care, support to and development of the health and care workforce and make better use of technology. All of these are covered in this book and these support our wider ambitions of preventing illness, tackling health inequalities and maximising the value gained for the taxpayers' investment in our NHS. We must all work together locally, regionally and nationally if we are to realise the opportunities of the NHS Long Term Plan and the associated investment.

People are living longer and are doing so with multiple co-morbidities (including multiple long-term conditions) and often as survivors of major health conditions that the NHS has helped them live through including cancer, cardiovascular disease and cerebrovascular accidents. Such complexity needs partnership and teamwork, partnership with patients and communities and teamwork across health and care. This will also require a greater understanding and engagement with patients and citizens that are empowered by greater access to information and ready access to technology, sometimes exceeding the access of their healthcare professional. On an individual level this offers opportunities of a paradigm shift in shared decision making. At a community level the fledgling primary care networks (PCNs) and integrated care systems (ICSs) offer the chance of greater engagement and shared solutions to long-standing challenges.

Primary care professionals have long-term relationships with patients, carers, families and often communities. The collaboration outlined in this book and supported by its case studies and exercises proposes that there is synergy in greater collaboration.

Changes to the general practice contract in the 1960s and 1990s saw the formation of group practices, employment of and then greater empowerment of general practice nurses (GPNs). The role of the GPN has become, like the GP, central to both proactive and responsive patient and population centred care. The new GP contracts in Scotland and England provide opportunities for adoption of a wider primary and community care workforce including pharmacists, social prescribing link workers, physician associates, paramedics and musculoskeletal (MSK) practitioners. These chapters focus on the considerable excellent development work such as developing clinical pharmacists as key members of the general practice team. Alongside all these new primary care roles, there is the development of advanced clinical practitioners (ACPs). General practice nurses, alongside others, are ideally suited to these ACP roles and as such this demonstrates ever more stimulating and rewarding career paths.

This book challenges us all to put aside interprofessional rivalries, to address differences in language and jargon to assure each other of mutual respect and trust, to support each other to work together and thus united to focus on providing the best service that we can for those we seek to serve. In so doing we ensure that together we meet the quadruple aim[3] of improving population health outcomes, individual experience of care, reducing per capita cost of care and improving the experience of providing care. Collaboration offers our best opportunity of achieving this aim. We hope that you will find this a useful resource to support system and care transformation.

Ruth May and Simon Gregory
April 2019

NOTES

1 Martin Roland, Barbara Starfield: An appreciation, *Brit Journal of General Practice* 2011; 61 (589): 523. https://doi.org/10.3399/bjgp11X588556
2 See https://www.longtermplan.nhs.uk/ [Accessed 21.5.19]
3 Rishi Sikka, Julianne M. Morath and Lucian Leape, The Quadruple Aim: Care, health, cost and meaning in work, *Brit Med J Quality and Safety* 2015. http://dx.doi.org/10.1136/bmjqs-2015-004160

Introduction

···

Sanjiv Ahluwalia, Karen Storey and John Spicer

We are delighted to present to you, the reader, with the wealth of knowledge of a wide range of professionals working in primary care. They have two things in common – a deep understanding of the power of primary care to improve the quality of people's lives and a passion for working together through collaboration – at its heart this book is about what that means and how to bring effective collaboration to life. Exactly who those healthcare professionals (HCPs) are will be described more fully through the course of the book, although for the moment we will mention doctors, nurses, pharmacists, paramedics and social work practitioners. Others will follow.

But you might ask, why is this important?

Like many of the developed healthcare systems across the world, we primary HCPs face an unparalleled challenge – how to maintain the quality of what we do in the face of increasing demands and fewer resources within which to do so.

Recognising this challenge, the National Health Service (NHS) in the UK has presented a blueprint called the Five Year Forward View (FYFV). The FYFV identifies the need for a blurring of boundaries between patients and the healthcare system, primary and secondary care, and physical and mental health. It has been recognised that breaking down these barriers will require collaboration between HPCs and patients, amongst HPCs across organisational boundaries, and between those that *commission* and organise healthcare and those that provide healthcare. But the FYFV does more than call for collaboration – it calls for collaboration to take place as close as possible to where people live, and communities can have a larger role in keeping people healthy and well – it calls for a renaissance in the provision of primary healthcare.

So the challenge our health economy, and those of others across the globe face, is how to enhance collaborative practice in primary healthcare as a means to enhancing quality and safety of care and patient and population outcomes, maintain or reduce the cost of healthcare provision, and make working in health a rewarding experience – often termed the quadruple aim by the Institute for Healthcare Innovation (IHI). We anticipate that this book will show you, the reader, how you can engage with this.

We have designed the book to support you through this journey.

In this book we define primary healthcare and its importance as well as collaboration with patients in primary care. We look at collaborative practice amongst professional in primary care and include examples from pharmacy, paramedicine, social care, and nursing. We consider the role of education in empowering the workforce to collaborate together as well as other enables such as commissioning and the role of technology in seeking to achieve the quadruple aim.

The workbook is in a format for readers to use in real-life situations as an opportunity to reflect and use their own experiences to think about collaborative practice. It can be used by students who are on a placement to consider the multi-faceted nature of collaborative practice in primary care and by those organising placements to ensure that they provide experiences that are meaningful and bring out the true value of collaboration. It is not a treatise on the theoretical and evidentiary aspects of collaborative practice – we have purposefully steered away from this to provide insights for students and practitioners alike. However, we infuse the whole book with references and key documents that the reader can pursue should they wish to know more. Although the book has a necessarily UK focus, we feel the account provided has importance for Europe and beyond.

We hope you find this book as valuable in your work and learning as we have in its development and shaping. Even if you do not read it from cover to cover, there is something in here to dip in and out of. This introduction would not be complete without thanking the many people (far too many to list here) who have been involved in its genesis – you know who you are; we thank you for this. Ultimately any mistakes of errors that appear in this workbook are ours and for which we take responsibility.

CHAPTER 1

Primary care: its modern context and the role of collaboration in practice

....

John Spicer

LEARNING OBJECTIVES

- Understand the meaning and challenges in primary healthcare.
- Appreciate why primary care is so important to patients, professionals and policy makers.
- Realise how primary care landscape links to collaborative care.
- Describe how UK primary care relates to other systems.

SO WHAT IS PRIMARY HEALTHCARE?

Trying to define primary healthcare (henceforward, primary care) is not easy. Whatever it is, the World Health Organization (WHO) considers it to be a good thing and the main method of delivering 'health for all', a key objective of the Alma Ata conference of 1978. This is significant as it places upon those of us who work in a primary care context a certain responsibility to work towards global health improvement – no small feat. We suggest that such aims cannot be delivered without interprofessional collaboration, whatever individual patient encounters may deliver. A quotation from that conference is worth considering:

> Primary health care is essential health care based on practical, scientifically sound and socially acceptable methods and technology made universally accessible to individuals and families in the community through their full participation and at a cost that the community and country can afford to maintain at every stage of their development in the spirit of self-reliance and self-determination.
>
> (World Health Organization 1978)

To return to the WHO context, five key features are ascribed to primary care:

- Reducing exclusion and social disparities in health (universal coverage reforms).
- Organising health services around people's needs and expectations (service delivery reforms).
- Integrating health into all sectors (public policy reforms).
- Pursuing collaborative models of policy dialogue (leadership reforms).
- Increasing stakeholder participation (WHO 2008).

These high-level objectives could be said to be the concern of policy makers rather than care deliverers, but they are worth holding in mind as we move on to consider what primary care is in its *actualité*.

EXERCISE

Consider the five high-level objectives listed.

- Does your health system organise its services around the needs of its citizens?
- If not, how would you change it such that it did?

Barbara Starfield, one of the greatest thinkers in this area, described the key characteristics of primary care as:

- Patients contacting their primary care service for all health-related needs.
- Care focussed on the needs of individuals (not around diseases – the domain of specialists).
- An orientation to individuals' family and community.
- Care provided for all health-related needs.
- Care provided in such a way as to ensure that all aspects are managed around the needs of the individual (Starfield et al. 2005; Shi et al. 1999).

From the patient or healthcare professional (HCP) point of view, if we attempt to unify these overarching descriptors, primary care is about the first contact between patient and professional, implying accessibility at point of need, a continuing duty of care and comprehensive and co-ordinated delivery. Generally such interactions take place in community clinics rather than highly technical institutions (even though in some countries there may be an overlap between the two). Given these rather general descriptors, primary care covers a wide variety of systems: from the 'barefoot doctors' delivering rural healthcare in the China of the 1960s and 1970s to the highly developed European primary care systems we have now (Friedberg et al. 2010; Smith 1974).

Previous research has demonstrated that the proportion of primary healthcare physicians in relation to the population is associated with better health outcomes for populations, whereas the proportion of specialists to the population appears to make little difference to health outcomes (Stange and Ferrer 2009). Whilst specialists are better at caring for people with a single disease, primary care physicians tend to be better at managing the care of patients with multiple conditions. Finally, those healthcare systems that have a greater orientation towards primary care tend to produce better outcomes for their communities.

Health systems with strong primary care thus produce better patient outcomes. Primary care also reduces the overall cost of healthcare to society. The ratio of primary care physicians to the population correlates well with the overall cost of healthcare (Franks and Fiscella 1998).

In the European system (e.g., exemplified mainly in the UK, Scandinavia and Holland) primary care has been founded on the work of medical generalists leading teams of HCPs and administrative staff who collectively deliver primary care to a registered list of patients. Certainly in the UK, that expert medical generalism is now extended to other healthcare professions: general practice nurses (GPNs) and clinical pharmacists, for example. They are the first point of contact for new illness episodes and take responsibility for preventative healthcare and (to variable extents) maternity, child health and chronic disease management. That a team of HCPs undertake such delivery of care requires collaboration amongst them – and we shall argue that care is immeasurably improved by that collaboration. Organisational arrangements can be relied upon for that delivery of care at first contact – and those arrangements can profoundly alter the degree to which collaboration is empowered or diminished. In a nutshell, then, this summarises primary care in its archetypal mode, and more detail will emerge in successive chapters.

WHAT DOES COLLABORATION IN PRIMARY CARE LOOK LIKE?

Case study

Peter attends a community clinic for care of his long-term gravitational ulcer. He sees a primary care nurse who regularly dresses this wound and also considers his general health and wellbeing. One afternoon his wound has deteriorated despite the nurse's attentions. It has become painful, sore and discharging. The nurse takes a wound swab for microbiological culture and checks other aspects of his condition. Not finding a cause for the deterioration, the nurse asks his colleague, a family physician, to assess Peter. After she has done this, they confer together and decide on a line of management, sharing the plan with Peter himself.

Consider what aspects of interprofessional collaboration are at issue in this case and how might it be fostered (Borrill et al. 2000).

This is an everyday example of two primary care professionals working together – simple but profound. The nurse is responsible for the continuing care of a patient, using his special skills of wound care, assessing for complications thereof and considering the wider implications of those complications. He is organising further necessary tests, which in this case may be assumed to need the intervention of secondary care-based laboratory services, and making a judgement as to the clinical importance of the patient's presentation. On the basis of that judgment, he asks a medical colleague to get involved as well, implying a need to access her diagnostic and management skills. Most importantly they involve the patient in the decision making around the problem before deciding on a plan. So, in response to the immediate need of the patient, they pool their skills and knowledge in his best interests. They probably know Peter over time and thus share a long-term understanding of his clinical needs. Thus they demonstrate a comprehensive, accessible and continuing response to Peter's acute and long-term needs. To get to the point that such care can be manifested, what should underlie that collaboration? The issues that might be included are as follows:

- *Mutual respect.* Both nurse and doctor should value their individual contributions to Peter's welfare.
- *Role understanding.* Both should understand their individual professional roles, although this might vary amongst different teams of HCPs.
- *Role adjustment.* Both should be prepared to vary their individual roles by mutual agreement and in their patient's best interests.
- *Shared values.* They should agree on the nature of the work they both do and how to do it for the better.
- *Organisational support.* Those who design the system within which both nurse and doctor work should do so with the patient's best interests at heart and their professionals' welfare within it.
- *Shared record keeping and IT.* This is a necessary adjunct to all of these issues.

This case is purposefully simple, involving only two members of the primary care team, but it illustrates key principles we seek to build on in future chapters.

The workforce of primary healthcare

Who then, more generally, are the HCPs who work in primary care and what sort of work do they do? It is important to review this area before considering how collaborative practice can work well. Primary care is the point of first access for UK patients, as is the case elsewhere, and the consultations that are engendered represent the vast majority of overall clinician-to-patient interactions. This order is purposefully not lexical, although reference should be made to the now historical role of the doctor delivering primary care more or less on his or her own. With good reason this has now been succeeded by a multi-professional team that is predominantly female.

Table 1.1 lists all the HCPs who work in UK primary care with their alternate titles.

TABLE 1.1 Healthcare professionals who work in UK primary care

- Practice Nurses, GPNs, Primary Care Nurses
- Physiotherapists
- Community Mental Health Nurses, Community Psychiatric Nurses
- Health Visitors, Children's Health Visitors
- GPs, Family Medicine Physicians, Primary Care Physicians
- Midwives
- Specialist Nurses (tissue viability, child protection et al.)
- Speech and Language Therapists, Speech and Language Pathologists, Speech Therapists
- Practice Managers, Business Managers
- Administrative Staff: Receptionists, Secretaries
- Pharmacists
- Pharmacy Technicians
- Paramedics
- Social Workers

EXERCISE

List the healthcare professionals in your team.

- Describe their working roles. If you don't know their roles, how can you find out about them?

Where such large numbers of professional roles are working, wholly or partially together, the scope for collaboration or indeed lack of collaboration is enormous. A further complexity is systemic and depends on the employer relations, payment systems and organisational structures. Again, to take the UK example, there can be many different employers who service these professionals in any given geographical area. This can include general practitioner (GP) practices, community health authorities, charitable and third-sector bodies, and even hospitals. Hospitals themselves can be subject to higher controlling bodies termed trusts or foundation trusts — these details need not concern us. Such complex employment arrangements can work against collaboration as we shall see.

Collaborative practice, more generally

Collaborative practice is not a new concept and has been widely discussed within the healthcare arena in relation to individual professional groups working together to improve the quality of care patients receive.

Collaborative practice may be defined as 'the continuous interaction of two or more professionals or disciplines, organised into a common effort, to solve or explore common issues with the best possible participation of the patient' (Bristol Royal infirmary 2001; Herbert et al. 2007).

Interprofessional education (IPE) provides a framework for collaborative practice, whereby it has been suggested that those who learn together work better together to improve patient care. It is distinguished from multi-professional education, where different professionals happen to be in the same learning environment – IPE brings professionals together to learn about each other's roles and develop an understanding of how each other's role may better help to improve patient care. That such professionals need to learn together to work together and thus improve individual and population health has been recognised at the international level by the WHO (1988).

Effective collaborative practice requires that those involved acknowledge and seek to understand the distinctiveness of each other's professional and developmental backgrounds and place these differences in the context of meeting the needs of patients. Once differences are explicitly acknowledged, these differences can be exploited to consider how individuals approach issues and practice with the aim of bringing about new ways of resolving problems. It is the combination of skills and knowledge that can be used to the best advantage to benefit patient care (Goto et al. 2018).

WHY IS COLLABORATIVE PRACTICE IN PRIMARY CARE IMPORTANT?

Primary care offers a unique set of challenges for any HCP and is different to the experience of collaborative working in other settings such as hospitals. Primary care practitioners tend to work in relative isolation in small teams with flat structures. By contrast, clinicians in hospital settings tend to work in hierarchical structures with larger teams. Primary care practitioners seek to form long-term relationships with patients for provision of chronic as well as acute conditions that can span several decades, whereas secondary care clinicians will provide episodic care for acute conditions. Secondary care services concentrate resources, tools and expertise within a small geographic and physical space (the structure of a hospital setting). By contrast primary care workers will need to link with several different organisations and types of HCPs in ensuring effective care for individual patients. The range of type of healthcare worker who may be involved in providing patient care also varies significantly between primary and secondary healthcare.

These differences in healthcare provision are not the only drivers for improving collaborative practice in primary care. Over the past decades, across the globe but particularly in some areas such as Europe or Japan, we are seeing an increasing number of people live longer and with more complex conditions. The ability of individual practitioners to care for people with multiple and often complex sets of healthcare needs is therefore challenged, with many reporting increased levels of stress and burnout (McKenzie-Edwards 2017). Sharing the challenge of increasing complexity and multi-morbidity with colleagues working in teams is therefore essential for patient and practitioner welfare.

THE POLICY CONTEXT

Many international agencies, including the European Union and WHO, have generated policy-related material to promote the development of interprofessional and collaborative practice. In the UK successive governments have produced and refined policy to support collaborative and interagency working.

The late 1950s saw the publication of the Younghusband Report (1959), which sought to improve interagency working amongst social workers and HCPs for the betterment of children and families. Throughout the latter half of the twentieth century, report after report called for improved collaborative working amongst different professional groups and agencies as a means of tackling safeguarding concerns.

The Bristol enquiry into the deaths of children undergoing cardiac surgery highlighted significant factors involved in the poor care of patients. These included poor communication, ineffective team working and professional silos where people did not work in the best interests of patients concerned. Lord Laming's (2003) investigation into the death of Victoria Climbié made the following specific recommendation:

> each of the training bodies covering services provided by doctors, nurses, teachers, police officers, officers working in housing departments and social workers should demonstrate that effective joint working between each of these professional groups features in their national training programmes.

In seeking to promote collaborative practice, government has developed a number of different approaches. These have included the ability of health providers to pool budgets and bring together diverse services under a single physical space.

National Service Frameworks (NSFs) for major conditions such as heart disease, diabetes and kidney disease were developed from the late 1990s to support the development of high-quality services and outcomes for patients. These NSFs (2001) were developed by multi-professional teams and made explicit reference to the need for collaboration amongst different professional groups with respect to delivery of care, communication and assessment of patients. The NSFs made reference to the need for professionals to engage with each other, patients and local communities to improve services and across traditional and non-traditional boundaries.

In the early 2000s Sir Derek Wanless was invited to view the future financial sustainability of the UK health system. A critical recommendation of his report was that to improve continuity of care for patients, members of the healthcare workforce needed to learn to work together. Further comment was made about viewing patients as 'co-worker' in their own care (Wanless 2004).

Given the serious concerns and repeated failures of agencies working in the arena of child safeguarding, government initiated multi-agency guidance based upon enacted legislation and a description of the roles and responsibilities of all agencies and professionals involved in the management of child safeguarding and welfare.

DOES COLLABORATING MAKE A DIFFERENCE?

There is an emergent evidence base on the benefits of collaborative practice for patients, HCPs and healthcare teams.

Patients receiving care from a collaborative primary care or community team have been shown to have better patient outcomes (Coventry 2014), reduced use of secondary and specialist services (Capp et al. 2017), improved concordance with healthcare advice and interventions and greater satisfaction with their experience of healthcare. The characteristics of high-functioning collaborative teams included clear objectives on the work they needed to undertake, with higher levels of participation from their team members, a strong focus on continually improving the quality of care and looking to develop new ways of providing care appearing to produce the most effective patient care (Morgan et al. 2015; Mulvale et al. 2016).

Furthermore, health workers have also reported improved job satisfaction and greater role clarity when working in teams by sharing problems and supporting each other (Taylor et al. 2001). The positive benefits of such teamwork included low levels of work stress and staff turnover.

CONCLUSION

We have offered a conceptual framework for primary care and a justification for the promotion of collaborative practice within it; and we contend that no rational or practical delivery of healthcare in the twenty-first century can be advanced without either of those things. In the rest of this book we will explore with examples and case studies how they might be achieved.

REFERENCES

Borrill, C. et al. (2000) *The effectiveness of health care teams in the National Health Service* report for DoH http://homepages.inf.ed.ac.uk/jeanc/DOH-final-report.pdf (Accessed 1.11.18).

Capp, R. et al. (2017) Coordination program reduced acute care use and increased primary care visits among frequent emergency care users *Health Affairs* 36 (10) www.healthaffairs.org/doi/full/10.1377/hlthaff.2017.0612 (Accessed 1.11.18).

Coventry, P. et al. (2014) Integrated primary care for patients with mental and physical multimorbidity: Cluster randomised controlled trial of collaborative care for patients with depression comorbid with diabetes or cardiovascular disease *BMJ* 2015: 350.

Franks, P. and Fiscella, K. (1998) Primary care physicians and specialists as personal physicians: Health care expenditures and mortality experience *Journal of Family Practice* 47 (2): 105–109.

Friedberg, M.W., Hussey, P.S. and Schneider, E.C. (2010) Primary care: A critical review of the evidence on quality and costs of health care *Health Affairs* 29 (5): 766–772.

Goto, M. et al. (2018) A cross sectional survey of interprofessional education across 13 healthcare professions in Japan *The Asia Pacific Scholar* https://doi.org/10.29060/TAPS.2018-3-2/OA1041 (Accessed 1.11.18).

Herbert, C. et al. (2007, August) Factors that influence engagement in collaborative practice: How 8 health professionals became advocates *Canadian Family Physician* 53 (8): 1318–1325.

McKenzie-Edwards, E. (2017) Professional self care in primary care practice: An ethical puzzle in *A Handbook of Primary Care Ethics* Papanikitas, A. and Spicer, J. Boca Raton, FL: CRC Press.

Morgan, S., Pullon, S. and McKinlay, E. (2016) Observation of interprofessional collaborative practice in primary care teams: An integrative literature *Review International Journal of Nursing Studies* 52 (7), July 2015: 1217–1230.

Mulvale, G., Embrett, M. and Razavi, S.D. (2016) 'Gearing up' to improve interprofessional collaboration in primary care: A systematic review and conceptual framework *BMC Family Practice* 17: 83 https://doi.org/10.1186/s12875-016-0492-1.

NSF for Diabetes (2001) https://assets.publishing.service.gov.uk/government/uploads/system/uploads/attachment_data/file/198836/National_Service_Framework_for_Diabetes.pdf (Accessed 1.11.18).

The report of the public inquiry into children's heart surgery at the Bristol Royal infirmary 1984–1995 (2001) *Learning from Bristol* CM 5207.

Shi, L., Starfield, B., Kennedy, B. and Kawachi, I. (1999) Income inequality, primary care, and health indicators *Journal of Family Practice* 48 (4): 275–284.

Smith, A.L. (1974) Barefoot doctors and the medical pyramid *British Medical Journal* 2: 429–432.

Stange, K.C. and Ferrer, R.L. (2009, July) The paradox of primary care *Annals Family Medicine* 1, 7 (4): 293–299 doi: 10.1370/afm.1023.

Starfield, B., Shi, L. and Macinko, J. (2005) Contribution of primary care to health systems and health *The Milbank Quarterly* 83 (3): 457–502 Blackwell Publishing www.commonwealthfund.org/usr_doc/Starfield_Milbank.pdf (Accessed 5.3.18).

Taylor, J., Blue, I. and Misan, G. (2003) Approach to sustainable primary health care service delivery for rural and remote South Australia *Australian Journal of Rural Health (2001)* 9 (6): 304–310.

The Victoria climbie inquiry: Report of an inquiry by Lord Laming (2003) *CM5730* www.gov.uk/government/uploads/system/uploads/attachment_data/file/273183/5730.pdf (Accessed 1.11.18).

Wanless, D. (2004) *Securing Good Health for the Whole Population* HMSO.

WHO (2008) www.who.int/topics/primary_health_care/en/ and *The World Health Report Primary Health Care: Now More Than Ever* World Health Organization www.who.int/whr/2008/08_contents_en.pdf?ua=1 (Accessed 1.11.18).

WHO Study Group (1988) *Learning Together to Work Together for Health* Geneva: WHO Technical Report Series No 769.

World Health Organization (1978) *Declaration of Alma-Ata* www.who.int/publications/almaata_declaration_en.pdf (Accessed 1.11.18).

Younghusband Report (1959) *Recommendations of the Younghusband Report 1959 on recruitment and training of local authority social workers* http://discovery.nationalarchives.gov.uk/details/r/C4957417 (Accessed 1.11.18).

CHAPTER 2

Collaboration with patients in primary care

....

Katie Coleman and Eleni Chambers

LEARNING OBJECTIVES

- Describe why it is important to support patients and take an active role in decisions about their health.
- Describe the key components of the collaborative care and the support planning model.
- Consider how patients and carers can become involved in the co-production of new services.

INTRODUCTION

This chapter aims to describe how patients and carers can collaborate in their own care in a primary care setting in the following ways:

- Ensuring they are supported to develop the necessary knowledge, skills and confidence to be active participants in their own care.
- The development of new services, using approaches of involvement and co-production.

This is not a comprehensive review of collaboration but will hopefully provide the reader with an insight to approaches that have been effective and may act as a springboard for greater exploration of other opportunities for collaborative practice.

The section on supporting patients and carers to take an active role in their own care is written with a focus on older people with greater complexity, people with long-term conditions (LTCs) and survivors of cancer (as LTCs) and will enable the reader to describe the process and skills required to deliver collaborative care and support planning (CCSP) for these cohorts of patients, consider possible barriers and solutions to implementing this approach at a practice, network and borough level, and provide examples of good practice and signpost to useful resources.

The section on co-production will take a broader look at collaboration with all registered patients and will provide the reader with a look at effective techniques used to date at both a practice level and wider. It will describe common barriers that may present and possible solutions and provide examples of good practice and signpost to resources that can be used to support future co-production opportunities.

Citizen participation has long been recognised as a component of democratic decision-making processes and recognises that involving people in their own care, as well as in the design and delivery of health services, is important. In September 1978, the Declaration of Alma-Ata was adopted at the International Conference of Primary Health Care. Not only did the declaration urge governments to commit to the delivery of primary healthcare for all, but it also promoted and declared it a human right for people to be able to *participate* as a group or individually in planning and implementing their healthcare. Yet collaboration continues not to happen uniformly, even though in medical practice, autonomy – that is, the ability of competent adults to make informed decisions about their own care through consenting to or informed agreement for any investigations or treatment – is considered a cornerstone of medical ethics and law.

COLLABORATION IN PRIMARY CARE: SUPPORTING PATIENTS AND CARERS TO TAKE AN ACTIVE ROLE IN THEIR OWN CARE

Why is it important to support patients and carers to take an active role in their own care?

We will all be patients or carers at some point in our lives and recognise when the interaction with health and care professionals is collaborative and person centred. Effective collaboration results in a partnership approach and ensures people feeling heard, informed and enabled to make the right choice. However, for many individuals this is not the experience they describe; they continue to experience care that fails to recognise that they are the experts about themselves (Tuckett, 1985) and that they possess the knowledge and skills that can provide invaluable insights to what's important to them as individuals and what will help them to make the right choices to improve their health and wellbeing. In addition, funding streams both for health and social care in England have failed to keep pace with increasing demand. To ensure the long-term sustainability of these systems, we need to consider a new approach that welcomes collaboration and recognises that patients who have the knowledge, skills and confidence to take an active role in their own care places fewer demands on services.

Society is changing; people are living longer in poor health, and there are now more than 15 million people with LTCs in England, whose care accounts for about 50% of all GP appointments and 70% of all inpatient episodes (Department of

Health, 2008; NHS England, 2015). In total, people with LTCs account for greater than 70% of the total NHS and social care expenditure, and as the number of people who live longer with LTCs is set to increase, these costs will rise accordingly in future years (Mathers et al., 2011). Yet, patients who are older with greater complexity and those with LTCs spend only a few hours with GPs or other HCPs each year and spend the majority of their time managing their conditions themselves, although the use of self-management does vary amongst conditions (Year of Care Programme, 2011; Chambers et al., 2015).

It therefore makes sense for the health and social care system to work with patients and carers, in collaboration, to encourage them to be informed and engaged, and so increasing their levels of activation, to facilitate them to manage their conditions to the best of their ability to ensure more effective utilisation of increasingly scarce resources. Activated patients (England, 2018) (this describe someone who has the knowledge, skills and confidence to manage his or her own health and care – this term is not universally liked and thus its use may be problematic), have been shown to have a lower utilisation of healthcare resources and is more likely to have a greater sense of control and to experience better health outcomes, including better mental health, reduced depression and decreased severity of symptoms (Coulter et al., 2015).

EXERCISE

Thinking about a consultation with a patient with LTCs:

● Discuss with a colleague how this contact could have been more collaborative.
● Why do you think this could have made a difference?

Where are we now?

For many years, policy makers, Royal Colleges, health charities and patients have called for greater involvement of patients in their own care to deliver person-centred approaches (NHS England, 2014a; Royal College of General Practitioners, 2014; National Voices, 2015; The Health Foundation, 2015), yet implementation continues to be limited. Across the NHS landscape, there are few incentives in place that encourage or promote person-centred care and effective collaboration with patients. General practice in England is currently incentivised to deliver disease-specific care through the Quality and Outcomes Framework (QOF) (Dixon et al., 2011), which rewards the delivery of a traditional medical model and fails to recognise the importance of a more psychosocial holistic approach, which encourages partnership working between healthcare professionals and patients. Furthermore, because people are living longer with greater complexity, the 'one size fits all' approach to consultation lengths in general practice isn't conducive to effective conversations that would support a collaborative approach to care (Flaxman, 2015).

NHS, Year of Care (Year of Care Partnerships, 2018), using the House of Care framework that support the implementation of a whole system approach to delivering person-centred care, has been providing support since 2007 to several sites across the NHS. The house, with its walls, roof and foundation acts as a metaphor, as well as a checklist, emphasising the importance and interdependencies of each element – if one element is weak or missing, the provision of person-centred care services are not fit for purpose.

EXERCISE

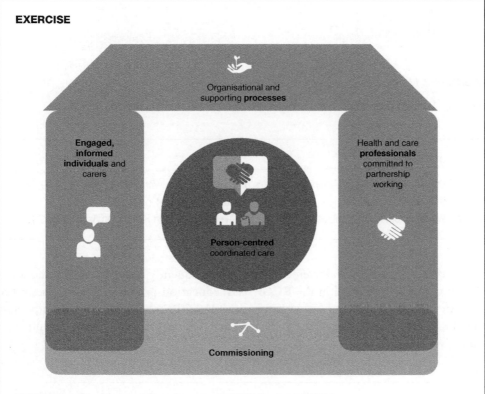

FIGURE 2.1 The House of Care framework (NHS England 2019b)

- What do the walls, roof and foundations elements of the House of Care framework represent?
- Using the House of Care framework, consider which resources and activities are in place within your practice that would enable collaboration with patients.

In June 2016, the Royal College of GPs (RCGP) endorsed a CCSP delivery model as a means by which GPs could deliver person-centred care in the context of the growing prevalence of multi-morbidity (Royal College of General Practitioners, 2018a). The CCSP model consists of six steps that ensures people are enabled to work in partnership with the health and care system so that they can become effective in self-management to address their own health and wellbeing needs (Royal College of General Practitioners, 2018b).

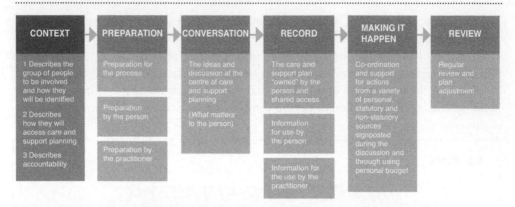

FIGURE 2.2 Model of care – collaborative care and support planning

Source: (Flaxman, 2015; Year of Care Partnerships, 2018)

EXERCISE

- Consider undertaking a mapping process of care for people with LTCs in your practice. Does it incorporate the six steps of personalised care and support planning?
- What systems would need to be in place to deliver CCSP (Helen Sanderson Associates, 2016)?

In response to this endorsement, it was subsequently agreed that the model of CCSP would be included in the RCGP's GP education programme and assessed as part of the RCGP membership exam. From 2019 GPs taking the membership exam will be expected to demonstrate that they have the knowledge, skills and confidence to deliver this approach.

EXERCISE

- Changing the conversation from 'What is the matter' to 'What matters' may help patients feel supported to consider what's important to them. With a colleague practice this approach.
- Are there other skills that would help you support patients to identify what actions they could take so they could do the things that are important to them?

Where do we need to get to?

In this section we will discuss the six elements of CCSP, looking at new ways of delivering this approach and new models of employment that may support general practice to deliver care to older people with greater complexity and people with LTCs. CCSP, as endorsed by the RCGP, aims to ensure practices take a systematic approach to the care of people with LTCs and multi-morbidity and build on the learning from Wagner's Chronic Care model (Wagner, 1998), the Year of Care Approach and Personalised Care and Support Planning as described by Think Local Act Personal (Think Local Act Personal, 2018). All these models of care recognise the importance of taking a planned, proactive approach to the care of people with complex health needs, offering holistic care through the involvement of multi-disciplinary teams and where working in partnership is central to care so that what is important to the patient is identified and addressed.

Case study: implementing chronic disease self-management approaches in Australia

England is not alone in identifying a need to take a more holistic person-centred approach to care. Across the globe, health and care systems are taking whole system approaches that recognise the challenges presented by people living longer with greater complexity.

In Australia patients with a chronic illness are offered a chronic disease management plan and/or a team care arrangements plan. The plans identify the patient's healthcare needs, specify the services to be provided by the GP and other health professionals, and outline the actions that the patient needs to take. A further standout feature of the Australian approach to chronic illness has been the recognition that the key to long-term population control of chronic illness is best obtained through modification of risk and protective factors underpinning their development and progression, such as the development of high blood pressure, obesity and high cholesterol.

A similar approach has been taken in Valencia, Spain, where Ribera Salud, has formed a public-private partnership, providing holistic person-centred care to patients over the age of seventy-five years with two or more LTCs. Central to this approach is the development of the complex care plan, which integrates medical care and social care and seeks to endorse patients and their carers as active participants in the care process. Key to this approach is the case manager/coordinator and the delivery of the agreed actions of the care plan (Australian Government, 2014; Browning and Thomas, 2015; McClellan and Gines, 2015).

Given that the needs of patients differ depending on their presenting issues, concerns and expectations, we need to recognise that the type of care offered cannot take a 'one size fits all' approach. Whereas the medical model, traditionally taught to undergraduate medical students and often used to manage acute episodes of care, ensures safe, effective care, but sees the patient as a recipient of care rather than a collaborator, for people with LTCs who spend most of their time caring for themselves, we need to ensure patients and carers feel engaged and informed by ensuring health and care systems provide them with the support to self-manage effectively and receive support tailored to their needs.

When patients are diagnosed with a LTC they will need varying levels of support from the outset. It is well-recognised that receiving a diagnosis of a chronic disease can have a profound effect on patients and their families' emotional and physical wellbeing (Diabetes UK, 2018). By referring patients to a care coordinator whose role may include helping patients understand their needs, supporting patient care activities between two or more service providers, addressing any underlying anxieties and helping identify their strengths at the point of diagnosis, patients may feel more supported to adjust to a new way of life that would then enable them to live well with their LTC and in turn prevent and delay the development of complications related to their diagnosis.

EXERCISE

● Increasing emphasis is placed on the provision of care coordination, but there is still confusion over its definition, what aspects of care it covers and what benefits it can deliver. Using the listed references, see if you can identify the answers to some of these issues (McDonald et al., 2007; Solberg, 2011).

Case study: American example of a care model employing care coordinators

The referral to a care coordinator is part of the core offer of the 'patient centred medical home' (Wagner, 1998; Think Local Act Personal, 2018), a US-based model of primary care based on Wagner's Chronic Care model, that has been able to demonstrate improved patient and provider experiences along with improved population health and has demonstrated reduced health costs and unnecessary service utilisation. The care coordinator role is seen as a crucial part of the model to ensure patients' needs are met and disease progression is prevented.

Once allocated, the care coordinator, in partnership with the patients and their carers, will ensure they receive regular reviews depending on their needs. This will help them stay well and prevent the development of complications related to their conditions.

Identification of a patient, at the point of diagnosis, who would benefit from a coordinated approach to CCSP will help maximise collaboration from the outset. However, due to the mobility of the population, it is important to establish an ongoing proactive approach to the identification of patients who would benefit from CCSP. This can be done at a practice level or, if data sharing agreements are in place, at a primary care network level or at a large-scale GP organisation level. It is important to ensure patients and carers are actively involved in co-producing any notifications around data sharing for direct care in accordance with the General Data Protection Regulations (GDPR) (EU General Data Protection Regulation, 2018; Londonwide Local Medical Committees [LMCs], 2018).

EXERCISE

● How does GDPR support greater collaboration with patients using health and care services?
● Undertake a review of the consent requirements introduced through GDPR (Australian Government, 2014; Browning and Thomas, 2015); discuss with a colleague what impact this may have on patient collaboration.

Having identified the context within which CCSP is to be offered, the next step is to ensure that the system, patients and carers, and practitioners and their associated teams are fully prepared for a CCSP conversation. Preparation may happen within an individual GP practice; however, as practices move towards working at scale with other general practice providers, there are opportunities of sharing patient data to develop care registries and so collectively undertaking planned care services together. This will help support greater coordination of care by centralising the call/recall systems, coordination of appointments, results, communications to patients and so on and will ensure patients and carers can get the right support, in the right place, at the right time. Not only will this be of benefit to the individual but also to individual practices that will experience the added value related to at-scale working.

Process preparation will take into consideration how a patient wants to be contacted, what the approach involves (what the patient should expect and what they will get out of this approach), and identify if any support is needed, if there is a preferred time for visits or tests and consent for sharing. A face-to-face clinical review should also be undertaken to collate baseline data for sharing with the patients so they are fully informed of their current health status. This should start with basic health checks, information that is currently collected as part of QOF to identify any issues that will help inform the CCSP conversation.

Individual preparation may involve receiving reflective prompts 'What's in it for me', self-assessment tools, peer-to-peer coaching support, identifying who they want to work with, receiving results in an accessible format and making an appointment for a CCSP conversation. Practitioner and team preparation may involve reviewing the patients' medical records, including medications, reviewing previous care plans and goals, identifying gaps in tasks or tests and making any appointments to address these gaps and consider what is and isn't working well from the practitioners' perspective. All these elements of preparation should be co-produced with patients and carers to ensure that the approach is person centred and addresses the needs of the local community.

Given that people's needs differ, health and care providers in collaboration with patients and carers should look to offer a more tailored approach to the care provided when preparing for a CCSP conversation. An example of this is the Quadrant Model for the management of LTCs, developed by Dr Ollie Hart, which utilises a patient's level of activation (Coalition for Collaborative Care, 2018). Using the patient activation measure (PAM) tool, repeated at agreed intervals of time, patients can be offered support that is tailored to their needs. It is recognised that this approach is still in its early stages of development and will need ongoing refining and new approaches to commissioning to ensure patients and carers are supported when they consider what approaches are available to them to improve their health and wellbeing. If effective, it is hoped that this approach will ensure more appropriate service utilisation and deliver greater capacity within the system so that the needs of patients, who have greater health and care requirements, are met.

Case study: a new model to encourage person-centred approaches to LTC management in primary care (the Quadrant Model)

In Sloan Medical Centre, Sheffield, they have been piloting an approach to develop self-management skills (patient activation) in people with LTCs, alongside normal clinical management. They started with patients living with diabetes and are looking to role this out to patients with other LTCs. Offering a CCSP approach, at the stage of preparation, a practice GP reviews the patient's results and notes and decides which of four quadrants the patient fits into (see Figure 2.3).

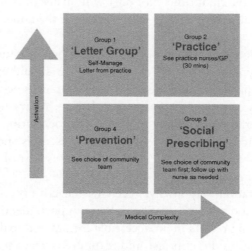

FIGURE 2.3 GP decision making depending on complexity (control) of condition and patient activation

Based on this review, Group 1 patients are sent a letter advising them that their diabetes is well-controlled and they appear to have a good understanding of how to manage their health issues. Group 2 patients are booked in for an extended (thirty minutes) follow-up appointment with a practice nurse or GP (or district nurse if housebound). A health coaching approach is used during these appointments, and all staff have been trained in this style of consultation. The appointment Groups 3 and 4 patients are contacted by the practice by telephone to check if they are happy to engage with a community team for their care and make a shared decision with the patient as to preferred provider. If patients have any concerns, they are offered an appointment to see a practice nurse. Of the patients referred to an agreed-upon community provider, the providers work with the assigned patients for up to three months and capture exit outcome measures (PAM + others specific to their service). All patients have their PAM, Hba1c blood test, lipids and BP check at six months. This model is in early stages of development, with the aim of being able to tailor care at scale.

Initial assessments are showing encouraging results, with a quarter of patients moving from Group 2 to Group 1. Nurses have expressed a preference to this way of working, and patients have also fed back, indicating that they are satisfied with the approach.

Another example that can help ensure patients are fully prepared for a CCSP conversation is peer coaching. This approach recognises that patients are often experts in their own conditions and can offer greater insight into the issues they are facing and can support people when considering how best to work in partnership with health and care providers.

Case study: a mental health peer coaching service developed by Cerdic Hall, mental health nurse consultant, Camden and Islington Mental Health Trust, in collaboration with Islington GP practices

The Mental Health Peer Health Coaching Initiative ran from January to April 2017 within Camden and Islington NHS Foundation Trust. It was a co-produced project, developed and delivered by HCPs and people with mental health problems. The purpose of the project was for primary care patients to receive up to three sessions of support from a peer coach, who also had experience with mental health problems. The aim was to help patients identify how to improve their physical and mental health. Peer coaches also worked with patients to complete a personalised care plan 'Snapshot', which was then shared with patients' GPs. Peer coaches attended training delivered by the Academy for Recovery Coaching to prepare for the role.

Key findings

Patients, peer coaches and GPs all recognised a need for peer coaching. Patients described how they were struggling with their mental health before participating, peer coaches felt that the standard support available does not meet the needs of people with mental health problems and GPs did not always feel they had the skill or capacity to work with people who have complex mental health needs.

The peer coaching project delivered benefits to all stakeholder groups. Patients could share their experiences with their peer coaches and felt listened to and understood. Some also reported wider impacts on confidence, connectedness, hope and clarity on how to achieve personal goals. For peer coaches, the role gave them a sense of achievement and improved confidence, inspiring some to pursue similar roles locally. For GPs, the main benefit was the information they received about their patients via the Snapshot. GPs also envisaged that peer coaching might help them manage their workloads, ensuring patients receive the support they need.

Once health and care providers, patients and carers have fully prepared for the CCSP consultation, a convenient time should be identified for both parties to address the patient's health and wellbeing needs. This should be an extended consultation in which a patient's goals are discussed through a collaborative conversation using shared decision-making approaches which are then documented in the patient's own words in an accessible format.

The importance of the holistic collaborative conversation has been recognised as central to the delivery of collaborative, patient-centred care. In New Zealand, an approach known as 'The Whole Person Approach' has gained significant recognition and describes how through effective conversations clinicians learn to deal with whole persons, recognising that the patient's story is a practical doorway into the complexity of the whole (Broom, 2016).

EXERCISE

- With a colleague take it in turns to identify an issue that you are currently experiencing and want to do something about. Through opening questions and active listening, attempt to identify goals that are important to you and will help you to start to address this issue. Write these goals down so you have a record of what you have agreed to do and to refer back to in the future. Remember to make your goals SMART (Specific, Measurable, Assignable, Realistic, Time-related) (Doran, 1981).
- Discuss with a colleague why it's important that care and support plan documents are recorded in a patient's own words.
- People access information in different ways due to differences in ability and preference. Find out about the NHS Accessibility Standards (NHS England, 2018a).

While documenting the CCSP consultation, patients should be supported to agree to a review date and to share this with their care coordinators who can then support the patients to achieve their goals. This support could involve the referral to a care navigator or a social prescribing link worker to help signpost the patient to local voluntary and community resources that would enable them to build on their personal assets and achieve their agreed goals. The *Marmot Review* identified that 70% of people's health and wellbeing needs are driven by social determinants, whereas only 30% are driven by clinical factors (Marmot and Bell, 2010). Voluntary and community-based services are well placed to support people's health and wellbeing needs, and by ensuring people are supported, through collaboration, to access these services, patients and their carers will be more able to increase their knowledge, skills and confidence to take more active roles in their own care, so reducing service utilisation as described earlier in the chapter (Year of Care Programme, 2011).

Case study: East Merton social prescribing pilot

Merton Clinical Commissioning Group (CCG) and Merton Council set out to test a model of social prescribing that would connect medical care with local voluntary and community resources. The Merton Voluntary Service Council social prescribing coordinator (SPC)/link worker delivered the pilot through two GP practices, Wide Way Medical Centre and Tamworth House Medical Centre, and the results were monitored for one year.

Key outcomes

- Patients self-reported health and wellbeing scores significantly increased between social prescribing visits (2.8 to 3.5; [$t(86) = 1.99$; $p = 0.00$]).
- Patients visited the GP significantly less in the three months after visiting the SPC than the three months before (11.9 to 8; [$t(137) = 1.98$; $p = 0.00$]).
- Patients visited A&E (Accident & Emergency) significantly less in the six months after visiting the SPC than the six months before (1.4 to 0.7; [$t(59) = 2.01$; $p = 0.04$]).

Conversations with patients and stakeholders alike showed that the pilot was highly valued and seen as a necessary service that filled a gap in local needs. Patients credit the programme to improving their wellbeing, bringing them back to recovery and linking them to support that is close to home.

What do we need to do to embed CCSP?

For the health and care system to effectively embed collaboration with patients and carers, we need to take a whole system approach as described by the House of Care. However, the challenge needed to support health and care professionals to adopt a collaborative approach cannot be underestimated. Developing the skills needed to work in partnership with patients and carers is essential and will need to be embedded in both undergraduate and postgraduate curricula, ensuring that people with 'lived experience' are supported to be part of the learning process.

Learning from new models of care and new national initiatives – for example, Integrated Personalised Commissioning (NHS England, 2017) – that look to create new relationships with patients and communities will help provide new opportunities for service provision that have collaboration at their centre (NHS England, 2014a).

Case study: Thomas and David's story

'My son is safe, healthy and happy – thanks to choice and control'.

Thomas Johnston, from Worcestershire, has profound and multiple learning disabilities. A personal health budget was used to fund 24/7 care and support for Thomas at an independent annex adjacent to his parents' home. Thomas's father David explains how the positive healthcare benefits for his son have been significant. The personal health budget has also resulted in the 'pendulum of power swinging to us', says David (NHS England, 2018b).

More evidence to support commissioning decisions is needed. The current body of evidence demonstrating that a 'more than medicine' or holistic approaches are effective (Horne et al., 2013) is growing; this in turn will support greater adoption.

However, the current approach to contracting does not encourage health and care providers to work together to take a holistic approach to patient's health and care needs. This will need to be addressed by organisations such as NHS Improvement and NHS England working collaboratively to change the NHS standard contract. In addition, there needs to be increased funding to the voluntary and community sector providers in recognition that the types of activities that address health and wellbeing of patients and carers are more frequently delivered by voluntary and community sector service providers.

Case study: a voluntary sector provider – Bengali Men's cookery session, Tower Hamlets (Year of Care Programme, 2011)

The need: traditionally, Bengali men are not engaged in cooking in the household so are not aware of ingredients in dishes. This makes it harder for them to understand how to eat healthily to better manage their diabetes.

The solution: Social Action for Health (SAfH), a local charity, was already engaged with Bengali men, helping them manage their diabetes. They employed staff from the local Bengali community, so language was not a barrier. They had access to kitchen facilities in a local, well-used community centre. SAfH engaged a local chef to run the cookery sessions and used their existing networks to recruit local Bengali men to the cookery club.

The provision and acquisition of knowledge is central to empowering patients and carers so enabling them to take a more collaborative approach with their health and care providers. As such there is a need for consistent and trusted information, delivered through a variety of approaches and accessible through recognised sources, which patients, carers and professionals can use. This may also be accessed through the voluntary sector, which can help disseminate information, deliver and promote self-management support programmes and offer prevention opportunities and engagement with local communities (NHS England, 2014b). Furthermore, Healthwatch, independent statutory organisations that act on the views of the public to improve local health and social care services, may assist with encouraging patients and carers to have a say in helping improve services and increasing people's knowledge and confidence in the process (Healthwatch, 2015).

Finally, access to electronic health records is important for patients, carers and professionals. For patients, their health data needs to be presented in accessible, understandable formats to assist with their participation. This includes access to records through a single portal, such as the NHS app, which will be available from all GP practices in 2019, rather than multiple portals currently on offer by the different providers. Professionals need to be able to share patient information, with patient consent, across all health settings so patients only need to tell their story once.

ENABLING PATIENTS TO COLLABORATE IN THE DESIGN AND DELIVERY OF CARE

Why is it important to enable patients to collaborate in the design and delivery of care?

Historically health services have been designed with the needs of the service provider in mind while failing to fully recognise or hear the needs of the patient. When collaborating in the design and delivery of services, everyone, including patients, communities, health and care providers and managers, should be recognised as having assets and bringing skills, abilities, time and other qualities to the process (Boyle et al., 2010b; Slay and Robinson, 2011; The Governance International Co-production Roadshows, 2011). By having this commitment to sharing power, a culture in which everyone is valued and respected and acknowledging the importance of diversity, accessibility and reciprocity, we can start to fully collaborate and co-produce health services (SCIE, 2018b).

Where we have failed to listen to patients and carers who use health services, we have seen unacceptable levels of care delivery, for example, The Stafford Hospital and Gosport Hospital scandals, and so to avoid future similar scenarios, we need to look at new ways to design and deliver services.

Collaboration through co-production provides this framework.

Work carried out by Nesta, a UK-based charitable organisation which focusses on relationships, states that 'people's needs are better met when they are involved in an equal and reciprocal relationship with professionals and others, working together to get things done' (Boyle et al., 2010a). This they describe as the underlying principle of co-production, which is comprised of the following key characteristics:

- Recognising people as assets.
- Building on people's existing capabilities.
- Promoting mutuality and reciprocity.
- Developing peer support networks.
- Breaking down barriers between professionals and recipients.
- Facilitating rather than delivering (Boyle et al., 2010a).

Demonstrating the financial impact of co-production is difficult, and even though there is some evidence that it can reduce costs, to date the available evidence is inconclusive (SCIE, 2018a). However, there is evidence of a range of other benefits and improvements. These range from improved service utilisation as a result of the insight people bring from their direct experience of services to greater social cohesion enabling the community to function more effectively (Shields, 2008).

The need to co-produce services has gained increasing importance over the years. In 2010 'The NHS White Paper, Equity and Excellence: Liberating the NHS' (Department of Health, 2010) included the aim of giving people who use services a stronger say, with more 'clout and choice in the system'; the term 'No decision about me, without me' was used to sum up this aspiration, although it had been used for some years by patients themselves prior to this.

This was followed in May 2014 by the Care Act, one of the first pieces of UK legislation to include the concept of co-production in its statutory guidance and, through joint working with local authority colleagues to integrate care, is beginning to impact on health service commissioning and provision through initiatives such as integrated personalised commissioning described earlier in this chapter.

Where are we now

As previously discussed, there are many useful and innovative examples of collaboration at an individual level, where patients and carers take active roles in their own care. These provide a diverse range of initiatives that can be learnt from and used in practice. However, when considering collaboration with patients and carers at a broader GP practice level, specifically in the design and delivery of primary care services, then collaboration is far less developed, and therefore the evidence base is lacking (Parsons et al., 2010; Sharma and Grumbach, 2017).

The most widely used approach for collaboration at this level are patient participation groups (PPGs) (Parsons et al., 2010; Smiddy et al., 2015). Since April 2015, it has been a contractual requirement for all GP Practices to have a PPG, although they have been in existence in some areas for much longer (Nagraj and Gillam, 2011). The National Association for Patient Participation (NAPP, 2018), is an umbrella organisation that provides support for such groups in primary care in the UK. They state that nearly all GP practices now have a PPG of some sort, with about 1,500 (approximately 20% of the total GP practices in England) affiliated to NAPP (Todd, 2018).

PPGs take many forms. Some groups meet face-to-face, and some are virtual; they have varied terms of reference, differing levels of support and involvement from GPs and other practice staff, and so on. The PPGs carry out a variety of functions, including the following:

- Being a critical friend to the practice.
- Advising the practice on the patient perspective and providing insight into the responsiveness and quality of services.
- Influencing the practice or the wider NHS to improve commissioning.
- Encouraging patients to take greater responsibility for their own and their family's health.
- Carrying out research into the views of those who use the practice.
- Organising health promotion events and improving health literacy.
- Communicating with the wider patient population.
- Running volunteer services and support groups to meet local needs.
- Fundraising to improve the services provided by the practice (The Patients Association, 2015; National Association for Patient Participation, 2017).

EXERCISE

- Consider what contextual factors may impact on the success of a PPG.
- Carry out a review of the approach your practice takes to run its PPG. Are there any factors that could be introduced to increase the patients' opportunities to be more involved in the design and delivery of services at your practice? Discuss these findings with colleagues and the PPG.

The diversity of PPGs is to be welcomed as it enables groups to respond to the needs of their local communities; however, this may make their development and facilitation more complex. In addition, the evidence for the effectiveness of PPGs is scarce, providing little robust research or evaluation to inform their growth and continued existence. The research that is available describes PPGs positively; however it also highlights possible difficulties with relationships with the practice team, in particular if the groups become 'too critical' and if the group focusses predominantly on one-off issues rather than providing ongoing strategic influence (Parsons et al., 2010; Newbould et al., 2015; Smiddy et al., 2015).

EXERCISE

- How would you go about setting up a PPG?

As individual practices start to work together more collaboratively to form primary care networks or large-scale GP organisations, there will be opportunities for PPGs to pool resources and work more collectively, particularly on those issues that are common to regions or boroughs.

It is suggested that PPGs are willing to contribute more effectively to service development, possibly by taking a stronger role in the commissioning process, but as with all collaboration activities, they need increased support and resources (Nagraj and Gillam, 2011; Newbould et al., 2015; Sharma and Grumbach, 2017). The following case studies provide some guidance for the development and support of PPGs.

Case study: Haughton Thornley PPG

Haughton Thornley PPG is a well established PPG located in Hyde, Cheshire. It has two main aims: to support the practice to deliver the best possible service and to promote good health for both patients of the practice and in the wider community. They carry out a wide range of activities to meet these aims, including the following:

- Facilitating a food bank.
- Providing workshops or talks on different issues, for example, on access to records, asthma or heart conditions.

- Working with other patient groups in the area on local or national concerns.
- Running stalls and raising awareness of issues in the local community, for example, for National Self-Care week or on dementia awareness.
- Consulting with patients to work on matters important to them and raising concerns over aspects of the practice.
- Liaising with the local CCG to provide feedback on relevant matters and to ensure the patient voice is heard.

They have regular meetings during which tasks are allocated, and interested patients usually work in teams on these and other issues when it is convenient for them as this enables more people to become involved.

More information, including a video about the group's activities, can be found here: www.htmc.co.uk/pages/pv.asp?p=htmc4.

Other examples of collaboration at this level are both scarcer and more localised. In addition, the use of different language to describe the initiatives increases the complexity, as will be shown.

The Altogether Better programme was established in 2008 and is described as a community-based approach that supports volunteers to carry out a range of 'Health Champion' roles within primary care (Altogether Better, 2018). These include facilitating groups such as for exercise, creative activities or peer support or assisting patients to use the practice better, for example, by helping with making appointments or checking in. An evaluation of the programme in thirty GP practices showed positive findings from both Health Champions themselves and other participants, including increased confidence, wellbeing and knowledge related to health. The majority of practice staff recommended the programme and valued the ongoing relationships with the Health Champions. Learning included the importance of selection and support of the Health Champions, the value of diversity and the challenges faced by working in an over-stretched NHS (McGregor et al., 2015).

In 2015 the King's Fund (2018) launched a national programme titled 'Leading Collaboratively with Patients and Communities'. Pairs, comprised of one health professional and one patient/carer, attended a five-day development programme that focussed on building collaborative relationships. The guide explores what helps to produce collaborative relationships and how embedding collaborative working can effect change in organisations, including within primary care (Seale, 2016).

CONCLUSION

Given that the provision of healthcare is all about the patient, it is easy to agree that morally, it is the right thing to do to ensure that care provided is done in collaboration with patients and their carers. As we have shown in this chapter, to achieve this requires changes at both the individual level in patients' own care and at a broader GP practice level in the development of new services. This wholescale change to current health systems needs resources and time to achieve. However, given that there is an increasing emphasis on this approach from policy makers, the introduction of CCSP into the curriculum for GPs and the increasing use of digital technology to share data, support self-care and ensure patients have access to reliable information, it feels as if we are starting to see some positive changes.

Further reading

Useful resources for supporting patients and carers to take an active role in their own care include the following:

1 www.england.nhs.uk/ourwork/ltc-op-eolc/ltc-eolc/house-of-care/
2 http://personcentredcare.health.org.uk/
3 www.rcgp.org.uk/clinical-and-research/resources/toolkits/collaborative-care-and-support-planning-toolkit.aspx
4 www.england.nhs.uk/ourwork/accessibleinfo/
5 www.health.gov.au/internet/main/publishing.nsf/content/mbsprimarycare-chronicdiseasemanagement

Useful resources for PPGs

1 Londonwide LMCs: www.lmc.org.uk/article.php?group_id=17111
2 NAPP [National Association for Patient Participation]: www.napp.org.uk/resources.html
3 The Patients Association: www.patients-association.org.uk/patient-involvement

Useful resources for other collaborations

1 The King's Fund, patients as partners. Building collaborative relationships amongst professionals, patients, carers and communities: www.kingsfund.org.uk/publications/patients-partners
2 The King's Fund, volunteering in general practice. Opportunities and insights: www.kingsfund.org.uk/publications/volunteering-general-practice
3 nef, Nesta, right here, right now. Taking co-production into the mainstream: www.nesta.org.uk/publications/co-production-right-here-right-now
4 NHS England, co-production resources: www.england.nhs.uk/participation/resources/co-production-resources/
5 NHS England, involving the public in primary care commissioning: www.england.nhs.uk/commissioning/primary-care/primary-care-comm/involving-the-public/
6 SCIE, co-production in social care. What it is and how to do it: www.scie.org.uk/publications/guides/guide51/what-is-coproduction/principles-of-coproduction.asp

REFERENCES

Altogether Better. 2018. *Altogether better* [Online]. Wakefield: Altogether Better. Available from: www.altogetherbetter.org.uk/home.aspx.

Australian Government. 2014. *Chronic disease management (formerly enhanced primary care or EPC): GP services* [Online]. ACT, Australia: Australian Government, Department of Health. Available from: www.health.gov.au/internet/main/publishing.nsf/content/mbsprimarycare-chronicdiseasemanagement.

Boyle, D., Coote, A., Sherwood, C. & Slay, J. 2010a. *Right here, right now: Taking co-production into the mainstream.* London: New Economics Foundation (nef), NESTA.

Boyle, D., Slay, J. & Stephens, L. 2010b. *Public services inside out: Putting co-production into practice.* London: nef, The Lab, NESTA.

Broom, B. 2016. Training clinicians in whole person-centred healthcare. *European Journal for Person Centered Healthcare*, 4, 402–408.

Browning, C. J. & Thomas, S. A. 2015. Implementing chronic disease self-management approaches in Australia and the United Kingdom. *Frontiers in Public Health*, 3, 162.

Chambers, E., Cook, S., Thake, A., Foster, A., Shaw, S., Hutten, R., Parry, G. & Ricketts, T. 2015. The self-management of longer-term depression: Learning from the patient, a qualitative study. *BMC Psychiatry*, 15, 172–186.

Coalition for Collaborative Care. 2018. *A new model to encourage person centred approaches to long-term condition management in primary care* [Online]. London: Coalition for Collaborative Care. Available from: http://coalitionforcollaborativecare.org.uk/tag/personal-centred-approaches/.

Coulter, A., Entwistle, V. A., Eccles, A., Ryan, S., Shepperd, S. & Perera, R. 2015. Personalised care planning for adults with chronic or long-term health conditions. *Cochrane Database of Systematic Reviews*, 1–131.

Department of Health. 2008. *Ten things you need to know about long term conditions* [Online]. London: Department of Health. Available from: http://webarchive.nationalarchives.gov.uk/+/www.dh.gov.uk/en/Healthcare/Longtermconditions/DH_084294 [Accessed 4/24/2008].

Department of Health. 2010. *Equity and excellence: Liberating the NHS.* London: Department of Health.

Diabetes UK. 2018. *Emotional wellbeing* [Online]. London: Diabetes UK. Available from: www.diabetes.org.uk/guide-to-diabetes/life-with-diabetes/emotional-issues.

Dixon, A., Khachatryan, A., Wallace, A., Peckham, S., Boyce, T. & Gillam, S. 2011. *Impact of quality and outcomes framework on health inequalities.* London: The King's Fund.

Doran, G. T. 1981. There's a SMART way to write management's goals and objectives. *Management Review*, 70, 35–36.

England, N. 2018. *Patient activation and PAM FAQs* [Online]. London: NHS England. Available from: www.england.nhs.uk/ourwork/patient-participation/self-care/patient-activation/pa-faqs/.

EU General Data Protection Regulation. 2018. *EU GDPR portal* [Online]. London: EU GDPR. Available from: www.eugdpr.org.

Flaxman, P. 2015. The 10-minute appointment. *British Journal of General Practice*, 65, 573–574.

The Governance International Co-Production Roadshows. 2011. *Transforming communities: Creating outcomes improving efficiency.* Birmingham: Governance International.

The Health Foundation. 2015. *Person-centred care resource centre: Self-management support* [Online]. London: The Health Foundation. Available from: http://personcentredcare.health.org.uk/ [Accessed 2015].

Healthwatch. 2015. *Healthwatch* [Online]. London: Healthwatch. Available from: www.healthwatch.co.uk [Accessed 2015].

Helen Sanderson Associates. 2016. *Progress in personalised care and support planning: Checking your progress in delivering personalised care and support planning.* London: Coalition for Collaborative Care.

Horne, M., Khan, H. & Corrigan, P. 2013. *People powered health: Health for people, by people and with people.* London: Nesta.

The King's Fund. 2018. *Leading collaboratively with patients and communities* [Online]. London: The King's Fund. Available from: www.kingsfund.org.uk/courses/leading-collaboratively-patients-communities.

Londonwide Local Medical Committees (LMCs). 2018. *GDPR: Further guidance now available* [Online]. London: Londonwide Local Medical Committees. Available from: www.lmc.org.uk/article.php?group_id=18482.

Marmot, M. & Bell, R. 2010. *Fair society, healthy lives: The Marmot review.* London: Institute of Health Equity.

Mathers, N., Roberts, S., Hodkinson, I. & Karet, B. 2011. *Care planning: Improving the lives of people with long term conditions.* London: Royal College of General Practitioners.

McClellan, M. B. & Gines, E. T. 2015. *Reinventing chronic care management for the elderly.* Washington, DC: The Brookings Institution.

McDonald, K. M., Sundaram, V., Bravata, D. M., Lewis, R., Lin, N., Kraft, S. A., McKinnon, M., Paguntalan, H. & Owens, D. K. 2007. Definitions of care coordination and related terms. In: Shojania, K. G., McDonald, K. M., Wachter, R. M. & Owens, D. K. (eds.) *Closing the quality gap: A critical analysis of quality improvement strategies.* Rockville, MD: Agency for Healthcare Research and Quality. AHRQ Publication No. 04(07)-0051-7.

McGregor, A., Hinder, S. & NMK Partners Ltd. 2015. *Altogether better evaluation report: Working together to create healthier people and communities.* Wakefield: Altogether Better.

Nagraj, S. & Gillam, S. 2011. Patient participation groups. *British Medical Journal (BMJ)*, 342.

National Association for Patient Participation. 2017. *What are PPGs?* [Online]. Surrey: NAPP. Available from: www.napp.org.uk/ppgintro.html.

National Association for Patient Participation. 2018. *Home page* [Online]. Surrey: NAPP. Available from: www.napp.org.uk.

National Voices 2015. *Care and support planning guide.* London: National Voices.

Newbould, J., Nagraj, S. & Gillam, S. 2015. "No point having a voice if no-one's listening": The views of members on the current and future challenges for patient participation groups. *Quality in Primary Care*, 23.

NHS England. 2014a. *Five year forward view.* London: NHS England.

NHS England. 2014b. *Future of health*, 11/21/2014. London: NHS England.

NHS England. 2015. *House of Care model: Background* [Online]. London: NHS England. Available from: www.england.nhs.uk/ourwork/ltc-op-eolc/ltc-eolc/house-of-care/ [Accessed 2015].

NHS England. 2017. *Interactive IPC operating model.* London, NHS England.

NHS England. 2018a. *Accessible information standard* [Online]. London: NHGS England. Available from: www.england.nhs.uk/ourwork/accessibleinfo/.

NHS England. 2018b. *Thomas and David's story* [Online]. London: NHS England. Available from: www.england.nhs.uk/personal health budgets/phbs-in-action/patient-stories/thomas-and-davids-story/.

Parsons, S., Winterbottom, A., Cross, P. & Redding, D. 2010. *The quality of patient engagement and involvement in primary care.* London: The King's Fund.

The Patients Association. 2015. Patient participation group information and support pack. Introduction and context. In: The Patients Association (ed.). Middlesex: The Patients Association.

Royal College of General Practitioners. 2014. *An inquiry into patient-centred care in the 21st century: Implications for general practice and primary care.* London: Royal College of General Practitioners.

Royal College of General Practitioners. 2018a. *Collaborative care and support planning* [Online]. London: Royal College of General Practitioners. Available from: http://rcgp-test.azurewebsites.net/clinical-and-research/our-programmes/care-planning.aspx.

Royal College of General Practitioners. 2018b. *Collaborative care and support planning toolkit* [Online]. London: RCGP. Available from: www.rcgp.org.uk/clinical-and-research/resources/toolkits/collaborative-care-and-support-planning-toolkit.aspx.

SCIE. 2018a. *Co-production in social care: What it is and how to do it: What is co-production: Economics of co-production* [Online]. London: Social Care Institute for Excellence. Available from: www.scie.org.uk/publications/guides/guide51/what-is-coproduction/economics-of-coproduction.asp.

SCIE. 2018b. *Co-production in social care: What it is and how to do it: What is co-production: Principles of co-production* [Online]. London: Social Care Institute for Excellence. Available from: www.scie.org.uk/publications/guides/guide51/what-is-coproduction/principles-of-coproduction.asp.

Seale, B. 2016. *Patients as partners: Building collaborative relationships among professionals, patients, carers and communities.* London: The King's Fund.

Sharma, A. E. & Grumbach, K. 2017. Engaging patients in primary care practice transformation: Theory, evidence and practice. *Family Practice*, 34, 262–267.

Shields, M. 2008. Community belonging and self-perceived health. *Health Reports*, 19, 51.

Slay, J. & Robinson, B. 2011. *In this together: Building knowledge about co-production.* London: New Economics Foundation (nef).

Smiddy, J., Reay, J., Peckham, S., Williams, L. & Wilson, P. 2015. Developing patient reference groups within general practice: A mixed-methods study. *British Journal of General Practice*, 65, e177–e183.

Solberg, L. I. 2011. Care coordination: What is it, what are its effects and can it be sustained? *Family Practice*, 28, 469–470.

Think Local Act Personal. 2018. *Personalised care & support planning* [Online]. London: TLAP. Available from: www.thinklocalactpersonal.org.uk/personalised-care-and-support-planning-tool/.

Todd, E. 2018. Personal communication with Eleni Chambers, 8 March.

Tuckett, D. 1985. *Meetings between experts: An approach to sharing ideas in medical consultations.* New York: Tavistock.

Wagner, E. H. 1998. Chronic disease management: What will it take to improve care for chronic illness? *Effective Clinical Practice*, 1, 2–4.

Year of Care Partnerships. 2018. *The house* [Online]. Northumberland: Year of Care Partnerships. Available from: www.yearofcare.co.uk/house.

Year of Care Programme. 2011. *"Thanks for the petunias": A guide to developing and commissioning non-traditional providers to support the self management of people with long term conditions.* Newcastle: Year of Care Programme.

CHAPTER 3

Organisations collaborating together

··

Sanjiv Ahluwalia

LEARNING OBJECTIVES

- Understand the role of collaboration amongst HCPs, with patients and amongst organisations.
- Appreciate the importance of accountable and integrated care to improve patient outcomes.
- Understand the shift towards integrated care in primary care.

INTRODUCTION

Earlier in this book we have considered the key characteristics of primary health-care which include patients contacting their primary care service for all health-related needs; care focussed on the needs of individuals (not around diseases – the domain of specialists); care with an orientation to individuals' families and communities; care provided for all health-related needs; and care provided in such a way as to ensure that all aspects are managed around the needs of the individual (Starfield, 1998).

In the UK, doctors trained as GPs provide primary healthcare. GPs traditionally work in local communities and are supported by a range of different workers including nurses, administrative staff and mental health and social workers working in teams. In the UK, traditionally general practice is the first port of call for access to healthcare. Primary care in the UK accounts for 90% of all initial contacts with the health system, the NHS (Parkin, 2018).

EXERCISE

Think about your family's use of primary healthcare and answer the following questions:

- What services does your primary healthcare provider offer?
- How do you think they could improve their service?
- How often have you needed to see someone outside of your primary healthcare provider?
- What challenges did you perceive in the interaction between your primary healthcare provider and others?

In the following sections, I shall explore some of the current approaches and ideas associated with collaborating with other professional groups within primary care and beyond; with patients as collaborators in their own health and wellness journey; and organisational collaboration that extends such thinking to include integrated care.

Collaborating with other professional groups

General practice is not the only occupational group in healthcare that has sought to undertake the journey to develop its professional identity. The last twenty years has seen the emergence of nursing, midwifery, and others seeking professional status and identity. These different groups have worked alongside each other and in constant interaction to maintain and develop their constructed identities and power relations. Within the sphere of community-orientated healthcare, GPs currently maintain a stranglehold (and power) on their work (through contractual and other mechanisms). However, the steady evolution of nursing, and the intervention of government policy to re-shape the dialogue amongst professional groups, has a direct impact on the nature and content of work undertaken by GPs. It has been suggested that nursing take on roles traditionally fulfilled by GPs (Sibbald, 2008), and evidence is emerging that nurses can undertake many of the activities of GPs with the same level of quality, at lower cost, and with higher patient satisfaction. GPs are increasingly expected to look after the more complex and challenging patients. The need for greater collaboration across professional groups has taken on a new urgency with a climate of economic austerity and against a policy framework that has resulted in fragmentation of services for patients.

Institutional support, equal status of participants and a co-operative ethos are the most important factors in developing successful interprofessional working and learning (Hewstone and Brown, 1986). Differences in history and culture amongst participants, interprofessional rivalries and differences in language and jargon as well as schedules and professional routines have been highlighted as barriers to successful interprofessional collaboration and education (Headrick, Wilcock and Batalden, 1998). There are also differences in regulations and accreditation of education, as well as differences in pay and status, which can be strong barriers to collaboration.

EXERCISE

- List out the groups of individuals from different professions that you work with.
- Which groups have you found it easy to work with and which have been more difficult?
- Are there other factors supporting interprofessional working that you can add to those mentioned in this chapter?

In considering the evidence for the benefits of IPE, Freeth et al. (2002) reported a systematic review of evaluations of such programmes. The authors identified fifty-three studies, most of which were about post-registration continuing development, based on workshops or short courses mostly from North America. The learning experience was always formal and of medium or long duration. Nursing and medicine were the most represented groups. Amongst the fifty-three studies, the authors found nine studies reported benefit to patients, fourteen studies improved cooperation and communication, twenty-one studies reported changes in organisational practice, twenty-four studies reported changes in knowledge and skills and twelve studies reported changes in behaviour. Five studies reported no change, and overall there were no negative comments.

Longer duration courses and those in the workplace are more likely to impact patient care and organisational and individual behaviours (Koppel et al., 2001). In addition, the maturity of the learner appears to influence outcomes. Studies focussed on continuing professional education reported changes in patient care and organisations, whereas studies focussed on pre-qualifying learners rarely had positive outcomes beyond the reaction and learning of the individual.

The evidence supporting interprofessional learning, however, is not without its critics. A Cochrane systematic review report (Reeves et al., 2017) failed to find any educational intervention meeting their required criteria of having robust experimental design and demonstrating benefit to patient outcomes. Knowledge of effectiveness is also limited because much of the literature is discursive. Few empirical studies have described the content of the interprofessional programmes, and the outcomes (educational or patient focussed) are poorly described or identified. The lack of rigorous evidence does not mean that IPE does not work. Nor should it be assumed that it supports the status quo. It is well recognised that the education of health professionals in the UK engenders discipline-specific norms and attitudes that act as a barrier with interprofessional collaboration (McPherson, Headrick and Moss, 2001).

Successful collaboration in teams benefits from time investment in developing shared aims and reflection to stimulate discussion across professional boundaries. Key competencies for individuals include the ability to describe their roles and responsibilities clearly to colleagues from other professions, recognising the constraints of that role and respecting the roles of others. So long as these competencies are present, practical problem-solving in collaboration with other professionals can provide opportunities for increased understanding, for example, by reviewing care of individual patients, introducing change to service provision and improving standards.

Collaborating with patients

The theory of cognitive dissonance (Festinger, 1957) describes the way in which uncomfortable feelings are experienced by individuals when confronted with contrasting perspectives. There is evidence that GPs experience these uncomfortable feelings in their interactions with patients (Ahluwalia et al., 2010; Odowd, 1988) and that these affect communication between doctors and patients. The issue of communication between HCPs and patients is of paramount importance to improved outcomes for patients and satisfaction with experiences of healthcare (Pollock, 2005). For example, misunderstandings between doctors and patients arose because of poor patient participation in shared decision making in consultations (Britten et al., 2000). Furthermore, in most of consultations, patients did not voice their agendas, and this led to consequences such as unnecessary prescriptions and non-adherence to recommended treatment (Barry et al., 2000). Despite nearly thirty years of UK government policy, educational approaches and consumer pressure to shift the balance of power within healthcare consultations, there remains a dominance of HCPs in the context of the consultation. Pollock (2005) highlights this thus:

> medical consultations continue to exhibit a structured asymmetry characterised by the passively and overtly differential demeanour of the patient and interactional dominance by the doctor.

It has been suggested that the ongoing predominance of doctors (and we can extend this to other HCPs) in healthcare interactions is a consequence of established patterns of interaction that seek to maintain the ability of both parties to 'save face' and prevent a breakdown to personal identity and self-esteem. Bureaucratic models of consultation are therefore used to perpetuate socially accepted patterns of interaction (Pollock, 2005) as they permit individuals involved to use strategies and tools that help in managing the dissonances created. Interactions between doctors and patients in the abstracted language of medical jargon, euphemisms, bureaucratisation of interactional process or inflated language (Lutz, 1989) can exclude patients from the resources, benefits and influence exerted to improve outcomes; whereas the inclusive interactions of acknowledgement of patient action and discursive space for communication offer the opportunity for doctors and patients to develop a common understanding of problems and search for therapeutic solutions.

Patients as experts in their own perspective was an idea introduced by Robert M Veatch (1991). It is part of a body of literature that has supported the development of collaborative practice between doctors and patients referred to as study of the consultation. Many researchers and authors have written about the consultation through the paradigm of the process (Byrne and Long, 1976; Pendleton and King, 2002), the role of participants (Veatch, 1991) and anthropological (Helman, 2004; Heron and

Group, 1989) and psychoanalytical approaches (Balint, 1957; Berne, 1964). Much of this literature has sought to achieve two things: re-dress the perceived imbalance in power relations between doctors and patients in consultations and bring forth the development of shared decision making and patient-centered care.

Recognising the potential for patients (as experts in their own illness and perspective) to take control of their own illness, policy in the UK has increasingly moved towards encouraging the concept of the 'expert patient' (Bodenheimer et al., 2002). Developing programmes specifically designed to empower patients to take active decisions about their own chronic disease is part of UK government policy and is increasingly seen in other parts of the world. Evidence from the UK and United States demonstrated that self-management programmes result in reductions in severity of symptoms, improved quality of life and improved communication between patients and doctors (Shaw and Baker, 2004).

A more recent innovation in the journey of patient empowerment has been the concept of personal healthcare budgets whereby patients are allocated a budget to use for purchasing the care that they might require. An evaluation of a three-year pilot programme highlighted that personal budgets for patients with chronic and LTCs improved quality of life for patients and their carers. Budgets were cost-effective for high-value budgets (i.e., greater than £1,000) and those patients with mental health issues or receiving long-term care (Forder et al., 2012). The NHS Long-Term Plan recommends a significant expansion of personal health budgets (NHS, 2019).

Organisations collaborating with each other

In previous sections, we have discussed collaboration amongst professionals and between professionals and patients in primary care. However, there is another form of collaboration in primary care worthy of mention – it is that of collaboration amongst organisations that provide care for patients in community settings. There has been an increasing recognition that patients suffer delays, they may have poorer outcomes and healthcare costs may rise because of poor or ineffective collaboration amongst organisations. Recent UK government policy has therefore turned towards identifying new ways of encouraging better collaboration amongst primary care organisations and beyond.

At the heart of recent activity has been the idea of integrated care as a means of improving patient outcomes whilst reducing healthcare costs through prevention of fragmented care and avoiding delays in communication and provision of care. General practice is particularly likely to benefit from integrated care approaches due to its interaction with many parts of the health and social care system. There are many definitions of integrated care reflecting the diversity of thinking and approaches (Shaw, Rosen and Rumbold, 2011). Integrated care may be defined this way:

> The patient's perspective is at the heart of any discussion about integrated care. Achieving integrated care requires those involved with planning and providing services to 'impose the patient perspective as the organising principle of service delivery.

Integrated care requires that the steps involved in a patient's journey through a diagnostic and treatment process are identified and, where possible, streamlined to reduce delays and improve efficiency. Suggested benefits have included converting guidelines into clinical practice, improving opportunities for data collation and audit, identifying areas within a care pathway where the quality of care may potentially be improved, as a means of encouraging more effective communication amongst professional groups aligned along an integrated care pathway, and reducing the burden associated with clinical records and their duplication by streamlining such processes. Commonly expressed concerns about integrated care approaches have been that patients will not receive the kind of attention necessary in a modern health system, complex or undifferentiated conditions are difficult to fit within the context of an integrated care system, and the linear approach to care planning engendered might stifle innovation and though such approaches may drive up quality they may have little or no impact on the costs of providing healthcare.

Integration amongst organisations can, broadly speaking, take two forms. One is where there is integration amongst organisations without significant clinical or service integration (horizontal); the other form is where clinical and service domains come more closely together into an integrated provision for patient care (vertical).

In 2009, the UK government initiated a number of pilots to test different approaches as a means of integrating care. Overall, these pilots reduced some outpatient and elective care but made no difference to emergency admissions (Roland et al., 2012). In November 2013, the Department of Health (DoH) in the UK, announced another fourteen sites for testing innovative approaches to integrating care and demonstrated that these new models of care reduced growth in emergency admissions relative to other areas and cites (NHS, 2019).

Integrated approaches to care provision are likely to fail unless the relationship between those engaged in the process of integration are able to work collaboratively (Barr, 2012). Improvements in communication at points of handover in a care pathway fail to convey the complexity of individual need and decision making that can only be fulfilled through an interprofessional, team-based approach to care delivery. Thus, integration of care processes requires an interprofessional underpinning, and vice-versa interprofessional teamwork can be enhanced through appropriate organisation of care services.

Based on current evidence, integrated care approaches show early promise in improving quality of care and influencing costs. There is concern that performance management approaches may distort the outcomes of care (Berwick, 2013; Francis, 2013). Wide commissioner–provider separation has also not yielded the expected levels of benefits. Current payment mechanisms for secondary care services in the UK follow a fee-for-service approach which encourages over-utilisation of services rather than coordination and integration of care. Indeed, this is an English phenomenon with the other countries (Scotland, Wales and Northern Ireland having abandoned such approaches). And although the capitated basis of primary care services are effective in keeping costs of service provision low (Starfield, Shi and Macinko, 2005), the opportunities for reducing costs are limited unless there is effective collaboration with secondary care to release savings to re-invest in local reform of services.

Accountable care

The combination of integrating care, reform of payment mechanisms and the sharing of risk is more likely to be successful in achieving the otherwise elusive goal of improving quality whilst reducing or abating healthcare costs. Consequently, a new form of organisational collaboration, the accountable care organisation (ACO) has emerged in the United States.

ACOs are collaborations of multiple provider organisations providing care to a defined population. They are accountable for achieving continuous quality improvement whilst seeking to reduce or stabilise costs. Primary care is a strong focus of all successful ACOs. There are multiple approaches to payment reform that arise in seeking to address the issues with current healthcare provision. These include providers sharing savings within a fee-for-service environment, extending the idea capitation as a limited or substantial part of the financial arrangements between commissioner and provider or moving towards agreeing that financial risk for poor-quality is absorbed by providers themselves.

Early evidence suggests that successful ACOs have a strong primary care orientation with a generalist focus around complex patient care (Ham et al., 2003) and are expected to meet a target framework focussed on patient-centred outcomes such as care coordination, population health outcomes, safety, patient engagement and utilisation of services.

There are multiple barriers to the development of ACOs including a lack of buy-in and understanding from providers fearful of losing autonomy and independence; lack of technical expertise (e.g., in establishing legal structures or adequate IT solutions); the absence of a supporting environment to help providers make meaningful quality and cost improvements; lack of cooperation from monopoly providers (e.g., large secondary care organisations with no interest in engaging with such payment reform); concerns about the risk to established service provision; and the potential complexity of any agreed pricing regime.

Early evidence, again from the United States, suggests that the ACO model can result in significant improvements in quality with modest cost savings (services). However, some providers have dropped out of the pilot programme in the United States due to the inevitable challenges (financial risk and service pressure) faced by this model.

PRIMARY CARE AND ITS JOURNEY TOWARDS INTEGRATED CARE

The last decade has seen a significant reconfiguration of secondary care services with fewer acute units providing more sophisticated care. At the same time, primary care has seen rising demand for services fueled by greater numbers of people living longer, shifting work from secondary to primary care, higher expectations of healthcare from better-informed patients, and higher levels of multi-morbidity. It is also being recognised that the trend towards higher workloads and demand is unsustainable especially in the context of a tight fiscal settlement for the NHS in the coming years. The current primary care workforce is under significant strain with GPs reporting high levels of emotional exhaustion (Baird et al., 2016).

These pressures have generated several policies that have sought to influence the provision of services in primary care. Lord Darzi (Darzi, 2008) first highlighted the need for GP and other community-oriented services to be co-located in polyclinics to capitalise on the potential for collaborative practice afforded through proximity. The RCGP (Lakhani, Baker and Field, 2007) offered the federated or networked model of clinical service delivery in primary care whereby practices in geographically contiguous areas could work collaboratively (sharing resources and best practice) in the development of new services. Networks and federations of practices are forming across the UK landscape. Internationally, federations or networks of community providers have thrived in New Zealand (Thorlby et al., 2012) and Canada. Clinical primary care networks can be seen as a response to the needs of service and clinical commissioners and are now being developed across England as part of the NHS Long-Term Plan.

Case study: developing collaboration across organisations in Tower Hamlets

The year 2019 marked the tenth anniversary of the formation of networks of practices in Tower Hamlets, aligned with local authority and local area partnerships. The drive for this was an acknowledgement that whilst access to good secondary care management of chronic diseases was less than optimal, care was also variable across primary care. The move of specific services from secondary care into primary care was accomplished by a funding shift that incentivised delivery based on commonly met Key Performance Indicators (KPIs); you were only as good as your least well performing practice in the network. There was some scepticism as to whether this would herald a 'race to the top or to the bottom', but the unpredicted and unintended consequence was that by working in partnership, if you were the less than optimally performing practice in a network, the incentive to improve, so as to not 'let the side down', kicked in. In addition, sharing of good practices and resources by others became natural. As well as a resource for delivering clinical care, the setup of networks involved funding of management structure and training. In terms of funding, a proportion of the annual monies was paid up front in advance, and a proportion was based on performance against agreed KPIs.

The next logical step came five years later when it became apparent that networks would need to come together as an entity to be in position to retain some of the services that they had been delivering when these were recommissioned. Bluntly put, despite having a track record of delivery, performance and care closer to home, each individual network was too small to get past stage one of the procurement process. Supported by the CCG, the Tower Hamlets GP Care Group was set up as community interest company in 2014 to represent all eight networks and thirty-seven practices within Tower Hamlets. This vehicle allowed GP providers to present 'one voice' at the table with colleagues in secondary care and social care in an integrated provider partnership. In addition, it was big enough as an entity to be able to bid for service contracts that were already being delivered by networks as well as to work together in partnership with others.

Having worked together collectively as individual organisations, Tower Hamlets Integrated Provider Partnership successfully applied for Multispecialty Community Provider Vanguard status in 2015 and as a partnership worked together to secure the community health services contract for Tower Hamlets in 2017.

CONCLUSIONS

Current arrangements for service delivery act against the development of integrated models of care capable of spanning traditional organisational and sector-related boundaries for the betterment of patients and local populations. The need to improve population health-related outcomes (a persistent failure of established health policy to date) requires an approach to care delivery that promotes integration between different parts of the health system and incorporates primary, community and social care. It also requires an emphasis on the values of local populations and their influence on the ways services are provided. The current education and training system is not designed to produce professionals skilled in the messy art of working across traditional boundaries, nor does current education equip healthcare workers to consider the needs of populations as well as individuals. There is an urgent need to enhance the generalist, collaborative and population-based skills of our healthcare workforce in primary and secondary care.

REFERENCES

Ahluwalia, S., Murray, E., Stevenson, F., Kerr, C. and Burns, J. (2010) '"A heartbeat moment": Qualitative study of GP views of patients bringing health information from the internet to a consultation', *British Journal of General Practice*, 60(571).

Baird, B., Charles, A., Honeyman, M., Maguire, D. and Das, P. (2016) *Understanding pressures in general practice*. London: King's Fund.

Balint, M. (1957) *The doctor, his patient and the illness*. London: Pitman Medical Publishing Company.

Barry, C. A., Bradley, C. P., Britten, N., Stevenson, F. A. and Barber, N. (2000) '"Patients" unvoiced agendas in general practice consultations: Qualitative study', *BMJ*, 320(7244), 1246–1250.

Berne, E. (1964) *Games people play the psychology of human relationships*. New York: Grove Press. Reprint.

Berwick, D. (2013) *A promise to learn: A commitment to act: Improving the safety of patients in England*. London: Department of Health, 6.

Bodenheimer, T., Lorig, K., Holman, H. and Grumbach, K. (2002) 'Patient self-management of chronic disease in primary care', *JAMA*, 288(19), 2469–2475.

Britten, N., Stevenson, F. A., Barry, C. A., Barber, N. and Bradley, C. P. (2000) 'Misunderstandings in prescribing decisions in general practice: Qualitative study', *BMJ*, 320(7233), 484–488.

Byrne, P. S. and Long, B. E. L. (1976) *Doctors talking to patients a study of the verbal behaviour of general practitioners consulting in their surgeries*. London: H.M.S.O. Reprint, NOT IN FILE.

Darzi, A. (2008) *High quality care for all: NHS next stage review final report*. London: Department of Health, pp. 1–92.

Festinger, L. (1957) *A theory of cognitive dissonance*. Stanford, CA: Stanford University Press. Reprint, NOT IN FILE.

Forder, J., Jones, K., Glendinning, C., Caiels, J., Welch, E., Baxter, K., Davidson, J., Windle, K., Irvine, A. and King, D. (2012) 'Evaluation of the personal health budget pilot programme'. https://www.phbe.org.uk/getFile.php?id=report. Accessed 13th April 2019.

Francis, R. (2013) *Report of the mid staffordshire NHS foundation trust public inquiry*. London: DH. https://webarchive.nationalarchives.gov.uk/20150407084231/http://www.midstaffspublicinquiry.com/report. Accessed 29th May 2019.

Freeth, D., Hammick, M., Koppel, I., Reeves, S. and Barr, H. (2002) *A critical review of evaluations of interprofessional education*. London: LSTN for Health Sciences and Practice, KCL.

Ham, C., York, N., Sutch, S. and Shaw, R. (2003) 'Hospital bed utilisation in the NHS, Kaiser Permanente, and the US Medicare programme: Analysis of routine data', *BMJ*, 327(7426), 1257.

Headrick, L. A., Wilcock, P. M. and Batalden, P. B. (1998) 'Continuing medical education: Interprofessional working and continuing medical education', *BMJ*, 316(7133), 771.

Helman, C. (2004) *Suburban shaman: A journey through medicine*. Cape Town: Double Storey Books.

Heron, J. and University of Surrey Human Potential Resource Group (1989) *Six category intervention analysis*. Surrey: University of Surrey, Human Potential Resource Group.

Hewstone, M. and Brown, R. (1986). Contact is not enough: An intergroup perspective on the 'contact hypothesis.' In M. Hewstone & R. Brown (Eds.), *Social psychology and society. Contact and conflict in intergroup encounters* (pp. 1–44). Cambridge, MA: Basil Blackwell.

Koppel, I., Barr, H., Reeves, S., Freeth, D. and Hammick, M. (2001) 'Establishing a systematic approach to evaluating the effectiveness of interprofessional education issues in interdisciplinary care', *Issues in Interdisciplinary Care*, 3(1), 41–49.

Lakhani, M. K., Baker, M. and Field, S. (2007) *The future direction of general practice: A roadmap*. London: Royal College of General Practitioners.

Battistella, E. (1991). 'Doublespeak: From 'revenue enhancement' to 'terminal living': how government, business, advertisers, and others use language to deceive you By William Lutz', *Language*, 67(2), 410–411.

McPherson, K., Headrick, L. and Moss, F. (2001) 'Working and learning together: Good quality care depends on it, but how can we achieve it?', *BMJ Quality & Safety*, 10(suppl 2), ii46–ii53.

NHS. (2019) The NHS long-term plan. London: NHS England.

Odowd, T. C. (1988) '5 years of heartsink patients in general-practice', *BMJ*, 297(6647).

Parkin, E. (2018) *General practice in England: Briefing paper*. London: House of Commons Library.

Pendleton, D. and King, J. (2002) 'Values and leadership', *BMJ*, 325(7376), 1352.

Pollock, K. (2005) *Concordance in medical consultations: A critical review*. London: Radcliffe Pub.

Reeves, S., Pelone, F., Harrison, R., Goldman, J. and Zwarenstein, M. (2017) 'Interprofessional collaboration to improve professional practice and healthcare outcomes', *Cochrane Database of Systematic Reviews*, 6.

Roland, M., Lewis, R., Steventon, A., Abel, G., Adams, J., Bardsley, M., Brereton, L., Chitnis, X., Conklin, A. and Staetsky, L. (2012) 'Case management for at-risk elderly patients in the English integrated care pilots: Observational study of staff and patient experience and secondary care utilisation', *International Journal of Integrated Care*, 12.

Shaw, J. and Baker, M. (2004) '"Expert patient": Dream or nightmare?', *British Medical Journal Publishing Group*, 328, 723.

Shaw, S., Rosen, R. and Rumbold, B. (2011) *An overview of integrated care in the NHS: What is integrated care*. London: Nuffield Trust.

Sibbald, B. (2008) 'Should primary care be nurse led? Yes', *BMJ*, 337.

Starfield, B. (1998) *Primary care: Balancing health needs, services, and technology*. New York: Oxford University Press.

Starfield, B., Shi, L. and Macinko, J. (2005) 'Contribution of primary care to health systems and health', *Milbank Quarterly*, 83(3), 457–502.

Thorlby, R., Smith, J., Barnett, P. and Mays, N. (2012) *Primary care for the 21st century: Learning from New Zealand's independent practitioner associations*. London, England: Nuffield Trust.

Veatch, R. M. (1991) *The patient-physician relation: The patient as partner*. Bloomington, IN: Indiana University Press.

CHAPTER 4

Learning to collaborate: boundary work and contemporary approaches in interprofessional education

....

Ann Griffin and Catherine O'Keeffe

LEARNING OBJECTIVES

- Revisit key concepts associated with education for collaboration including multi-professional and IPE.
- Be introduced to the emerging concepts of trans-professional education, hybridicity, border discourse, related educational theories and their value for understanding professional identities as context change.
- Consider the importance of educational relationships for promoting collaborative learning across primary, community and integrated care settings.
- Identify essential components when designing educational programmes for collaboration.

BACKGROUND

There is increasing focus on the need for professionals to be able to work effectively in multi-professional teams (Imison and Bohmer 2013). Collaborating is considered crucial to respond to the complex needs of patients with LTCs; the emergence of new, diverse roles with varying degrees of professional status; and systems and structural re-organisation within the NHS. Failures in education to respond to the changing needs of the population, to persist with hospitals as the preferred educational setting and a lack of focus on teamwork and leadership are now the focus of global educational reform (Frenk et al. 2010). However, a significant barrier to progress is 'the so-called tribalism of the professions – that is, the tendency of the various professions to act in isolation from or even in competition with each other' (ibid). There has been much discussion on the value of interprofessional learning, an educational model which supports improved collaboration and its contribution to better healthcare (see, e.g., Clifton, Dale and Bradshaw 2006; Faresjo 2006 and Barr and Low 2013). IPE, learning 'with, from and about each other' (Barr and Low 2013), is widely regarded as an essential educational strategy to break down siloed thinking and working to develop professionals who have the skills to be effective collaborators and team members. Effective teamwork requires each professional to have some understanding of the nature of the roles and professional identities of other team members. However, the impact of context also has an important influence on professional identities and how they are expressed within teams. Of increasing importance is the need for educators to work and support learners collaboratively across settings as integrated care pathways are promoted in response to community and primary care focussed service development (NHS England 2014).

Multi-professional education was described by Barr and Low (2013, and expanded in the CAIPE statement of 2017) as

> occasions when professions learn side by side. Interprofessional education is defined as occasions when professions learn with, from, and about each other, to improve collaboration and the quality of care.

Rather than a mixed professional group learning to perform the same skill or acquire specific knowledge, IPE focusses on sharing professional perspectives and expertise to understand the roles and working practices of the other – to understand *how* to work collaboratively. Trans-professional education takes our understanding of collaboration one step further. It has a more holistic view of healthcare collaboration and includes '"non-professional" health workers e.g. ancillary staff, administrators, managers, policy makers, community leaders' (Frenk et al. 2010). Trans-professional education thereby permits a 'systems approach' examining the practices and processes of healthcare systems but equally mindful of individuals' professional boundaries and roles – both traditional and emerging (Thistlethwaite 2012).

In this chapter we will illustrate the pressing need to educate for collaboration in primary and community settings. We will begin by considering the professional roles now emerging within this setting and discuss opportunities as well as the tensions involved in learning to collaborate. We will focus on IPE and supervision as this is an area of critical importance. We will then briefly examine a range of literatures, including theoretical, that help educators develop a more nuanced understanding of education for collaboration. We will then present a case study from London which exemplifies some important features of educating for collaboration within this context.

THE CHANGING NATURE OF THE MULTI-DISCIPLINARY TEAM

Frenk et al. (2010) in the Lancet Commission, *Health Professionals for a New Century: Transforming Education to Strengthen Health Systems in an Interdependent World*, advises educators to promote interprofessional and transprofessional education that breaks down professional silos while enhancing collaborative and non-hierarchical relationships in effective teams . . . develop[s] a common set of values around social accountability.

(p. 1924)

The need for educators in primary care to work collaboratively and interprofessionally is becoming more pressing given the emergence of expanded and new roles across a range of HCPs. Five Year Forward View (FYFV) and subsequent reports, including the Roland Commission on Primary Care (Roland 2015), have identified trends including a growing ageing population with complex comorbidity and LTCs and the move to 'personalised medicine' informed by developments in genomics as well as technological innovation which require a move away from approaches to treatment and care based on 'one size fits all'. Current and future health professionals will need to retain and develop generalist as well as specialist skills and the ability to adapt throughout their careers to accommodate new and expanded roles. Such capabilities are essential to ensure that flexible services are provided that can respond to emergent patient and population needs. The King's Fund (2015) summarises these challenges noting:

The workforce of the future needs to be able to take on a greater breadth of tasks to meet increasingly complex patient needs, while working across different care settings and multidisciplinary providers. The challenge for the health service is to ensure that there is sufficient staff for current models of care, while also moving towards this very different future.

(p. 4)

Recent education reviews, including the 'Shape of Training' (Greenway 2018) and 'Shape of Care' (Willis 2015), have highlighted approaches to health education that need to be adopted to prepare both the current and future workforce to respond to these challenges. In primary care, responses are being developed based on the recommendations of these reviews. Health Education England (HEE) is supporting training for advanced clinical practitioners (ACPs) in primary care including supporting GPNs to access advanced training to develop their capacity to assess patients and prescribe. NHS England (NHSE, 2017) have introduced a national programme to implement expanded pharmacy roles within GP practice as a key approach to improving the quality and safety of service delivery across the primary care system. Both the advanced training of GPNs and the introduction of clinical pharmacists in primary care represent expanded roles for existing HCPs. Physicians associates (PAs) are also being deployed in primary care. The PA is an example of a new role – the practitioners perform specific medical functions under the supervision of a doctor. PAs are usually science graduates who have completed a two-year postgraduate programme. Currently they are unregulated, although they can join a voluntary register hosted by the Royal College of Physicians. The emergence of changing and new roles raises the question of how education needs to develop to prepare all practitioners to understand and work effectively across a wider range of professionals with varied responsibilities and scope of practice. Collaborative approaches to education are emerging to respond to these challenges.

EXERCISE

Consider the clinical or educational teams you work with.

- In what ways are the roles of team members changing?
- Are there any new roles within these teams?
- How are changes in roles or the emergence of new roles impacting on professional identities and educational needs?

EDUCATION AS THE PREDOMINANT DETERMINANT FOR COLLABORATIVE LEARNING

Education has been positioned centre stage as the mechanism that supports collaborative learning: 'It represents the principal lever for promoting collaborative values amongst future healthcare professionals' (Martín-Rodrígues et al. 2005). In this next section we discuss commonalities in IPE including the development of supervisors and curricula before moving on to highlight the barriers which undermine inter professional education interventions.

All of the roles mentioned in the previous section of this chapter require supervision and support from educators working in primary care which can present significant challenges, not least supporting the development new emergent professional identities. The significance of the effective supervision for workplace learning has been re-emphasised in the Francis report (Francis 2013), the NHS Education Outcomes Framework (DoH 2013b) and the DoH Mandate to Health Education England (DoH 2013a). Consequently, educators are increasingly required to consider flexible, collaborative, interprofessional approaches to supervising learners in clinical practice. Arguably this should be a relatively straightforward process, as research (Austerberry and Newman 2013; Bentall 2014) has shown that the domains that underpin the frameworks and guidelines for clinical teachers are very similar. All refer in different ways to, for example, the need to focus on facilitating learning using appropriate learning theories, creating a safe and supporting learning environment and assessing and evaluating learning. Common themes regarding requirements include education as a requirement of all practitioners, reference to protecting patients and balancing local flexibility with the benefits of national standards of quality. Such commonality suggests that there are opportunities for collaboration across professions even if entry requirements for clinical teachers from specific disciplines are more restrictive.

Being equally prepared for multi-disciplinary or multi-professional work is featured across health professionals' curricula and occurs in one form or another across most of the professions. Interestingly although preparing learners for multi-professional work is mentioned in most of the documents reviewed, only a few areas actually stress the idea of interprofessional or shared learning. These include nursing, healthcare science and some of the allied healthcare professions, such as podiatry. Such programmes may have modules that are taught interprofessionally or learning activities such as interprofessional group activities.

Despite our unified goal to enhance patient care, our shared educational mission and common vision as espoused in curricula, collaborative work can be hard to achieve. There are a range of reasons for this relating to organisational and structural issues as well as individual factors. Bringing together learners is often a logistical challenge; working professionals as well as healthcare students are often geographically separate. Putting on a programme of education that is meaningful for all professionals, permitting equal contribution and benefit, also tests the skills of interprofessional educators. A common concern that can inhibit interprofessional approaches to supporting workplace learning in healthcare is the position that individual health professions are distinctive and learners need to learn in different ways, which would make teaching them together difficult. An alternative, more expansive view is that reflection on clinical context can be harnessed to recognise that roles and boundaries may become blurred, creating new legitimate opportunities for collaborative learning. However, there has been no systematic investigation into how learning is perceived within each professional area and whether in fact there are great differences.

Individual factors include the power and hierarchy differences that can work to reinforce stereotypes and marginalise other professionals (Martín-Rodríguez et al. 2005; Floyd and Morrison 2014). In Baker et al.'s (2010) research professionals were seen to preserve their own sense of identity when involved in IPE, which acted as a barrier to shared decision making.

Others go further and urge us to take a more critical lens to the concept of IPE (Floyd and Morrison 2014). They wish to counter the assumption that 'being professional today means being interprofessional' (Hammick et al. 2009, p. 37) and the unquestioned supposition that this form of education leads to better patient care.

EXERCISE

Reflect on your experiences of teaching and learning with other professionals.

- What similarities have you noticed in curricula and in approaches to teaching and learning?
- What are the main differences?
- In what ways have professional identities and power relations helped or inhibited sharing and learning?

THEORETICAL PERSPECTIVES: CONTACT HYPOTHESIS, 'PROFESSIONAL PROJECTS' AND 'HYBRIDICITY'

In this section theoretical approaches are described that can help in understanding common barriers to IPE and collaborative learning. IPE is often criticised for being under-theorised, without sufficient explanatory frameworks for the clinical educator to understand why certain approaches to IPE succeed or fail (Floyd and Morrison 2014; Paradis and Whitehead 2018; Reeves et al. 2017). These theories focus on the influences of stereotyping and power in creating boundaries and in helping understand ways in which the educator can influence these social barriers and support the renegotiation of professional identities and values.

Contact theory is the most frequently used theoretical framework for IPE (Paradis and Whitehead 2018). It is based on the work of Allport (1975), who explored the negative effects of stereotyping on intergroup race relationships. He found that interpersonal contact and learning about the other group decreased prejudice by promoting understanding of the different cultural norms and values. However, in order for contact theory to work effectively, the groups must be of equal status, they should have a common goal and prestige and rank should be minimised. These later reasons explain why poorly constructed IPE often only reinforces negative stereotypes and leads to educational initiatives failing (Paradis and Whitehead 2018).

Traditional professional education reflects what Larson (1977) describes as 'professional projects', whereby occupational groups are seen to work towards utilising social stratification for their own advancement. Macdonald (1995) examines how this concept has been used to study the rise of professionalism in an extensive review of research on the sociology of the professions. Macdonald (1995) argues that traditional professions, such as law and medicine, are awarded higher social status and rewards by virtue of their specialist knowledge and control and highly competitive entry to the profession. In this model the professions are seen to be autonomous in terms of determining who enters the profession, how they are educated and trained and ultimately how they gain power for autonomous practice. Aligned occupational groups in healthcare, such as nursing or the allied healthcare professions in this model are deemed to have 'semi-professional' status as their ability to practice autonomously is constrained by the more dominate professional group, in this case, medicine. Occupations with semi-professional status may aim to emulate established professions by introducing higher entry requirements and more academically demanding training programmes as well as attempting to produce a distinct body of knowledge to support their practice (Macdonald 1995). However professional projects are active phenomena (Larson 1977). Professions constantly react and adapt to changing circumstances to maintain, and improve, their own social and economic capital. Their strategic (re-)positioning reveals either professional advancement or regression. Changing professional roles such as the increased autonomy of ACPs and the emergence of new roles such as PAs embody the re-positioning of professional projects in practice. Underpinning this re-positioning is the struggle over the control of 'boundaried' specialist knowledge and consequently areas of professional practice. This struggle can also be the source of interprofessional tension and conflict, creating a challenging and contentious space for educators to work in.

In recent years emerging models of professionalism have been identified that may help educators approach their work in contentious, boundaried areas. Whitty (2008) values more collaborative and democratic models of professionalism that recognise the socially constructed nature of the healthcare disciplines[1] and the need to challenge established boundaries between professionals in practice and the education of those beginning their professional careers. A key driver for challenging the established models of traditional professionalism is their reliance on what are seen to be unique bodies of knowledge that inform specialist professional practice, practice that aims to address specific issues or problems. Such specialist approaches are however unable to address the issues and challenges that arise as a result of the 'complexity' and 'super complexity' associated with current professional life (Barnett 2008). The so-called wicked problems that professions are required to attempt to solve cannot by their very nature be addressed by one discipline. Rather strategies are required that enable professionals to recognise the many different factors that influence the problems professional practice aims to address. In healthcare such complexity is evident on many levels, from the range of drugs and treatments that individual patients may require to the social factors that influence the support available to aid recovery.

A contemporary theory of IPE therefore needs to facilitate flexible interpretations of roles and professional identity. Greenwood and Maanaki Wilson's (2006) developed a theory of 'hybridicity'. Hybridicity refers to the work practitioners do when they broker different sorts of disciplinary knowledges. Hybrid practitioners act as in-betweeners, actively engaging with these different knowledges, re-contextualising and co-constructing knowledge which can be integrated and applied to practice. This co-construction of knowledge permits new opportunities for identity and role but also exposes new conflicts and threats. However, a key feature of the hybridisation of knowledge is to blur traditional professional boundaries, see Whitchurch (2008). Making the demarcation of professional knowledge less certain and more changeable allows for emergent, expansive professional projects. Professional narratives under these circumstances can become less bounded and encourage a 'border discourse' (Perloff 1998), promoting a reflective and expansive notion of professionalism.

EXERCISE

Consider one or two complex issues in your professional practice that may not have clear solutions and which by their nature require collaboration across disciplines to care for patients.

- Can you identify examples of underpinning knowledge regarding patient care that is blurred, less certain and not confined to one professional group?
- If so, what educational challenges and opportunities can arise when you are supporting teaching and learning on these issues?

Current research exploring the impact of changes in traditional roles, the emergence of new roles on professional identity, and collaborative practice that would help our understanding of border discourse and implications for educational support and supervision is limited. The evaluation of the Programme for Integrated Child Health (PICH) is an example of an educational intervention aimed to nurture the development of collaboration. What follows is a summary of a formal evaluation which illustrates the affordances of this educational space.

Case study: learning to collaborate – the Programme for Integrated Child Health

PICH was established by paediatricians at Imperial College and St. Mary's hospitals, London, in 2014. PICH is an intraprofessional education programme for trainee paediatricians and GPs supporting them to set up, deliver and evaluate integrated care across primary and secondary care. Over a year-long course, trainees work together on integrated care projects for children, with the skills that they learn by doing so augmented by monthly training seminars and mentoring from senior clinicians with experience in developing integrated care systems.

The evaluation involved interviews with programme mentors and previous trainees and observations of teaching sessions aimed to explore the effectiveness of the programme. The participants highlighted the persistence and prevalence of rigid roles and boundaries in operation in healthcare environments. Silos were reported as commonplace. Notably, education and training were reported as contributing to this situation, as a PICH mentor reports, 'The vast majority of the people they'll train in a medical school or a nursing school – stay in one place and never get out of the four walls'. So traditional educational systems, which promote immersive socialisation, contribute to establishing barriers to collaboration (Martín-Rodríguez et al. 2005).

However, by coming together in the PICH, participants, whilst retaining a clear sense of professional identity, were able to change their attitudes and behaviours. By understanding their own roles and those of others more clearly, they were able to develop enhanced collaborative practice. Building effective relationships and communication was key to traversing chasms that prevented professional collaboration. As one trainee reports,

> The primary care . . . aspect . . . that's been really important. And I'd argue it matters less about what the actual content is than getting those multiple lenses. Because what you start to experience then is how multiple views on a particular situation can completely unlock things. And what my hope is that people start taking that into other aspects of their working lives.

This was not just between doctors but within healthcare teams, including patients. Relationships and communication were strengthened by mutual dialogue and sharing stories. The educational space provided by the PICH was fundamental to this learning as another trainee illustrates:

> Hearing the discussions between GPs and paediatricians has been really interesting. You know there's often a grey area between what's in the realm of GP and what's in the realm of the paediatrician but is actually lots of shared work and this actually lots of unknown areas that we just sort of fudge through.

This finding mirrors the work of other research highlighting the central importance of communication and relationships (Martín-Rodríguez et al. 2005; Suter 2009).

However, workplace spaces were more problematic and acted as barriers to collaborative practice through varied and changing structures and systems. This coupled with the individual factors – rigid professional identity, boundaried specialised roles and stereotyping – highlights the struggles *in action* that occur in workplace settings. Further research is needed into how the principles revealed in the PICH evaluation could be applied more broadly and result in growing impact on clinical settings. However, the evaluation gave tentative cause for optimism and demonstrated how educational environments could encourage collaboration.

EXERCISE

Reflecting on the experience of the PICH programme, consider whether you may be able to apply some of the approaches they developed to training initiatives you are involved in or whether you could consider different approaches that would enable learners to gain greater insight into the roles of other professionals to promote collaboration in practice.

CONCLUSION

Traditional approaches to professional education in healthcare are being challenged to prepare practitioners to work collaboratively and flexibly across professional boundaries as health systems adapt to emergent population healthcare needs. IPE has, with varying degrees of success, attempted to promote collaborative working across the healthcare professions. In this chapter we have argued that IPE needs to be re-positioned as collaborative education that promotes reconstructed hybrid professional identities (Whitchurch, 2013) through border discourse and boundary working if it is to enable educators to create innovative strategies ensuring learners become capable and confident practitioners in this changing context. Educational theories discussed in this chapter provide intellectual tools educators can use to engage their professional imagination (Powers 2008) to think and act differently as they design and implement new, innovative educational programmes as exemplified by PICH. The example shared demonstrates how a carefully crafted educational programme can enable learners to develop new insights into their own professional identities and that of others. Such insights challenge traditional siloed perspectives on practice as learners engage in border discourse on the grey areas of practice that may be seen as complex, difficult and challenging. Reflection on learning through border discourse can enable learners to understand the value of and develop the skills needed to practice collaboration for the benefit of patient care. A key attribute of such programmes is collaborative education, which provides opportunities to develop interprofessional relationships and to renegotiate how professional identities are enacted mindful of contemporary healthcare practice.

The complexity of contemporary clinical practice situated within systems that are changing rapidly – socially, culturally and structurally – affects professional education (Martín-Rodríguez et al. 2005). For collaborative education to be effective Paradis and Whitehead (2018) note that attention needs to be paid to structural and external factors:

> In overemphasizing education, we ignore the systemic issues that underpin problems of collaboration. Future education for collaboration should stress the limited impact of educational interventions when trying to solve major structural problems and ensure that organizational and legal factors are included as essential areas for improving collaborative care delivery.
>
> (p. 1461)

Although little empirical research has been undertaken in this area, Martín-Rodríguez et al. suggest that consideration needs to be given to the organisational structure and philosophy in which educational programmes are developed. Time and space for collaborative learning in situ needs to be planned for and supported by the organisation providing learning opportunities – all of which have implications for the commissioning and financing of education. Due consideration will be required of these broader organisational and contextual factors if education for collaboration is to succeed.

Education for collaboration is a complex and challenging field. The educational theory and practice we have reviewed suggest that essential components need to be considered as educational programmes are designed most notably:

- They should ensure there are opportunities for learners to work and engage in meaningful discussion with professionals and learners from a variety of disciplines to provide opportunities for border discourse – such opportunities need to be accompanied by reflective discussion with educators to promote insight into collaborative professional practice.
- Educators need to develop their leadership skills to create safe spaces where learners and clinicians working with them in practice can feel comfortable discussing professional identities and boundaries, both traditional and emergent. Such spaces can help reduce a sense of professional protectionism that may inhibit open discussion of ways practitioners can work across established boundaries.
- Educators need to recognise the opportunities and constraints associated with specific organisational contexts. Working with educational commissioners, due consideration needs to be given to social, cultural and structural factors that could impede learning so that educational programmes can be crafted to provide time and space to ensure collaboration and aid learning.

As educators develop expertise in designing collaborative education in response to shifting contextual affordances, it is possible that fluid hybrid professionals become the 'valued' professional currency. That being interprofessional becomes synonymous with collaboration, understanding interprofessionality and advocating interprofessional supervision and education as a means of promoting interprofessional learning may represent an emergent hybrid collaborative professional practice. Professionals who work and learn in collaborative, interprofessional ways could help practitioners formulate appropriate values in difficult situations as they can be more flexible about how they see their professional selves and understand their roles and partnerships.

NOTE

1   Disciplinarity in this context refers to regulated professions within healthcare, for example, medicine or nursing.

REFERENCES

Allport, G.W. (1975) *The nature of prejudice* (25th Anniversary Edition). Reading, MA. Addison-Wesley.

Austerberry, H. and Newman, M. (2013) *Review of qualifications and training for clinical educators in the healthcare professions*. London. Social Science Research Unit, Institute of Education, University of London.

Baker, L., Egan-Lee, E., Martinmianakis, M.A. and Reeves, S. (2010) Relationships of power: Implications for interprofessional education. *Journal of Interprofessional Care*, 25(2): 98–104.

Barnett, R. (2008) Critical professionalism in an age of supercomplexity. In Cunningham, B. (Ed.) *Exploring professionalism*. London. Bedford Way Papers: 190–208.

Barr, H. and Low, H. (2013) *Introducing interprofessional education*. Fareham. CAIPE.

Bentall, C. (2014) *Study and the views on teaching and learning within health qualifications in England*. London. HENWL.

Centre for the Advancement of Inter Professional Education (2017) Interprofessional education guidelines, Barr, H., Ford, J., Gray, R., Helme, M., Hutchings, M., Low, H., Machin, A. and Reeves, S. Available: www.caipe.org/resources/publications/caipe-publications/caipe-2017-interprofessional-education-guidelines-barr-h-ford-j-gray-r-helme-m-hutchings-m-low-h-machin-reeves-s [Accessed 24.2.19].

Clifton, M., Dale, C. and Bradshaw, C. (2006) *The impact and effectiveness of interprofessional education in primary care: A literature review*. London. Royal College of Nursing.

DoH (2013a) *The department of health mandate to health education England*. London. Department of Health.

DoH (2013b) *The education outcomes framework*. London. Department of Health.

Faresjo, T. (2006) Interprofessional education: To break boundaries and build bridges. *Rural and Remote Health*, 6: 602. Available: www.rrh.org.au/journal/article/602.

Floyd, A. and Morrison, M. (2014) Exploring identities and cultures in inter-professional education and collaborative professional practice. *Studies in Continuing Education*, 36(1): 38–53.

Francis, R. (2013) *Report of the Mid Staffordshire NHS Foundation Trust public inquiry*. London. The Stationery Office.

Frenk, J. et al. (2010) Health professionals for a new century: Transforming education to strengthen health systems in an interdependent world. *The Lancet*, 376(9756): 1923–1958.

Greenway, D. (2018) *The shape of training*. London. The General Medical Council.

Greenwood, J. and Manaaki Wilson, A. (2006) *Te Mauri Pakeaka: A journey into third space*. Auckland. Auckland University Press.

Hammick, M., Freeth, D., Cooperman, J. and Goodsman, D. (2009) *Being professional*. Cambridge. Polity Press.

Imison, C. and Bohmer, R. (2013) *NHS and social care workforce: Meeting our needs now and in the future*. London. The Kings Fund.

The King's Fund (2015) *Workforce planning in the NHS*. London. The King's Fund.

Larson, M. (1977) *The rise of professionalism: A sociological analysis*. London. University of California Press.

Macdonald, K. (1995) *The sociology of the professions*. London. Sage.

Martín-Rodríguez, L.S., Beaulieu, M.D., D'Amour, D. and Ferrada-Videla, M. (2005) The determinants of successful collaboration: A review of theoretical and empirical studies. *Journal of Interprofessional Care*, 19(sup1): 132–147.

NHS England (2017) *Next steps on the Five year forward view*. London. NHSE.

Paradis, E. and Whitehead, C. (2018) Beyond the lamppost: A proposal for a fourth wave of education for collaboration. *Academic Medicine*, 93(10): 1457–1463.

Perloff, M. (1998) Cultural liminality/aesthetic closure?: The 'interstitial perspective' of Homi Bhabha. In Bhabha, H.K. (Ed.) *The location of culture*. London. Routledge: 139–170.

Powers, S. (2008) The imaginative professional. In Cunningham, B. (Ed.) *Exploring professionalism*. London. Bedford Way Papers: 144–160.

Reeves, S., Pelone, F., Harrison, R., Goldman, J. and Zwarenstein, M. (2017) Interprofessional collaboration to improve professional practice and healthcare outcomes. *Cochrane Database of Systematic Reviews*, (6). Art. No.: CD000072. DOI:10.1002/14651858.CD000072.pub3.

Roland, M. (2015) *The future of primary care: Creating teams for tomorrow*. London. HEE.

Suter, E., Arndt, J., Arthur, N., Parboosingh, J., Taylor, E. and Deutschlander, S. (2009) Role understanding and effective communication as core competencies for collaborative practice. *Journal of Interprofessional Care*, 23(1): 41–51, DOI:10.1080/13561820802338579.

Thistlethwaite, J. (2012) Interprofessional education: A review of context, learning and the research agenda. *Medical Education*, 46: 58–70.

Whitchurch, C. (2008) Shifting identities and blurring boundaries: The emergency of third space professionals in UK higher education. *Higher Education Quarterly*, 62(4): 377–396.

Whitchurch, C. (2013) *Reconstructing identities in higher education: The rise of the third space professional*. London. Routledge.

Whitty, G. (2008) Changing modes of teacher professionalism: Traditional, managerial, collaborative and democratic. In Cunningham, B. (Ed.) *Exploring professionalism*. London. Bedford Way Papers: 28–49.

Willis, P. (2015) *The shape of caring: Raising the bar*. London. Health Education England.

CHAPTER 5

The role of technology in collaborative primary care

....

Ruth Chambers and Marc Schmid

LEARNING OBJECTIVES

- Understand the relevance of underpinning LTC care with technology-enabled care services (TECS) in primary care.
- Realise that collaboration is essential for shared care management across primary care teams and with clinicians in other healthcare settings that include TECS set up along LTC pathways and overseen by responsible clinicians.
- Be confident that you can design and set up at least one mode of digital delivery of care in your general practice, collaborating with other practice team members and clinicians in other health settings who share responsibility for providing care for your patients.

HOW ARE THINGS NOW?

Adoption of TECS is a complex process with a minority of front-line teams across all healthcare settings embedding technology into their day-to-day work, with vast numbers of practitioners and patients being left behind. As a result, technology is often deployed in ad hoc ways, with its real purpose never being realised. We suggest a need to identify and overcome barriers that exist to deployment of TECS and promote ways to overcome such challenges and speed digital transformation of TECS in primary and community care front-line settings at scale (Chambers et al. 2016).

A positive and supportive organisational culture is essential to underpin the adoption of digital delivery and requires transformational change. To achieve that we need evidence of the benefits of different modes of digital delivery at scale across primary care in collaboration with staff in other healthcare settings. The evidence for the extent to which remote care effectively supplements or underpins or replaces face-to-face care still remains to be seen.

Solutions must be able to demonstrate measurable health and/or economic benefits in the context of clearly identified needs. Where solutions are proven to add health or financial benefits, their adoption should be part of mainstream, commissioned health services and move away from dependence on project funding as quickly as possible.

UK primary care is undergoing significant pressures – at a level never experienced before. Demand is increasing, and the need for collaboration underpinned with the adoption of technology is more important than ever. However, technology alone is not the answer. For technology to succeed primary care teams need to be confident and skilled enough to fully realise the benefits and willing to collaborate along LTC pathways. E-clinicians should be envisaged as the norm who are confident and competent in their understanding and use of digital modes of delivery so that patients are engaged and involved in their healthcare management. Such e-clinicians who drive change successfully will be of different levels of seniority in a wide range of clinical specialties and have personal qualities such as resilience, persistence and collaboration as well as being willing to listen, learn and then adapt their everyday provision of digital care.

EXERCISE

Consider where you are in relation to digital literacy and ownership.

1   Which of the following statements most closely describes how you feel in relation to using digital technology as part of your practice?

- *'Digitally Worried'*: I am nervous about using digital delivery of care for patients.
- *'Digitally Ready'*: I feel comfortable with using digital modes of delivery and have the know-how and skills to adapt to the changes.
- *'Digitally Leading'*: I see the opportunities on offer, and I am a champion for the adoption of digital healthcare.

2   Which of the following statements do you agree with? Digital technology, data and information used in healthcare will

- make a large, positive contribution to self-care or shared management of patients with LTCs in the community.
- make a small, positive contribution to self-care or shared management of patients with LTCs in the community.
- make no difference or even have a negative impact on self-care or shared management of patients with LTCs in the community.

ORGANISATIONAL PERSPECTIVES OF TECS

Organisations need health economy-wide agreements for enhancing collaboration amongst healthcare teams with wide-scale availability and interconnectivity of TECS embedding its use as part of usual service delivery. These agreements must mitigate the current overall fragmentation in England amongst health, social care and public health services by introducing a shared integrated healthcare record system with agreed interoperability standards and ownership. (Other UK countries may be more easily moved to common TECS as that fragmentation is not so obvious.) In that way practice staff will have shared access to hospital, community and maybe social care patient records. Clinicians need to be confident that information they access about a patient in such an integrated care record is accurate and up to date and that access by clinicians and organisations is underpinned by information governance agreements relating to collaborative work amongst different health and social care teams.

There is potential to develop an area-wide network of digital clinical champions who can drive collaboration between settings and should in time be able to deliver substantive cost, clinical and quality benefits by using pre-determined modes of TECS for patients or carers/citizens in relation to LTCs or lifestyle habits. They might share responsibility for the delivery of digital care with clinicians in other health or social care settings in a real-time basis, or pass on or take on responsibility for the digital delivery of care for a specific patient to a clinician based in another healthcare organisation or share responsibility across their practice team – as Figure 5.1 shows. These modes of digital delivery include the following:

- Increased use of social media to support patients with LTCs.
- Improved access to service operation by patients (e.g., booking appointments or requesting repeat prescriptions in general practice) and intelligent use of GP Online.
- New modes of consultation in line with the GP Forward View (NHS England 2016).
- Reduction in proportion of face-to-face consultations by general practice clinicians and patients based at home or in a nursing home, for example, substitution by video consultation or telemedicine.
- Adoption of online consultation platforms designed to reduce demands on practices as team members triage patients' relaying of symptoms and requests.
- Increase in access to self-care information and then shared management of LTCs, for example, via Flo simple telehealth interactive text messaging between clinician and patient and between clinicians in primary care with those in other healthcare settings (see Figure 5.1 and case study).
- Consistent professional approach to recommending or using trusted apps by clinicians in primary care and other front-line settings across the health economy.
- Web-based multi-disciplinary team video conferencing meetings for primary care teams within and across healthcare organisations.

1 Shared real-time responsibility: by primary care clinician and at least one other clinician/social worker from different healthcare organisations/settings and share TECS directly (same mode of technology or connected if different) for delivery of shared care plan of same patient/same condition at same treatment phase (clinicians/social workers have agreed responsibility via care plan).

2 Shared sequential responsibility: by primary care clinician and at least one other clinician/social worker from different healthcare organisations/settings interface, so one hands over responsibility to the other for providing TECS directly (same mode of technology or different) for continuing care of same patient/same condition via agreed care plan. (This might be by general practice nurse defining the patient pathway and endorsing the TECS protocol for others to provide with real-time support e.g., advice in person/by email.)

3 Shared multidisciplinary protocol with one TECS operator: by primary care clinician and at least one other clinician of different discipline, in same general practice or practice group, sharing (delegated) responsibility for providing TECS directly (≥ one mode of technology) for continuing care of same patient≥ one condition via agreed care plan. (This might be by general practice nurse defining patient pathway and endorsing TECS protocol for others to provide with real-time support e.g., advice in person/by email.)

4 Self-contained delivery by individual professional: TECS initiated and delivered by primary care clinician who updates other health/social care professional(s) or teams involved in amongst patient's care (i.e., giving information rather than interactive decision making amongst professionals). It might be that a patents requested the inclusion of their personal technology such as an app in their care that the initiating practice nurse has adopted.

5 Patient-driven and provided: patient has collated bodily measurements from dependable source such as FitBit watch or home blood pressure machine, then brings to practice nurse to add to patient's records and update progress of agreed care plan.

FIGURE 5.1 Five-level framework for extent of responsibility for delivery of TECS by primary care clinicians and other health and social care professionals (each level assumes that the patient/service user has given informed consent to participate and that it may be one or more health conditions or any digital health modes of delivery provided)

Such deployment of digital modes of delivery of care should match national priorities for effective healthcare usage such as the following:

- Improved medication adherence through better communication and reminders.
- Reduction in numbers of did not attends (DNAs) in primary and community care and other healthcare settings.
- Better integrated care record sharing so that history taking is only done once, minimising duplication of investigations and reducing the likelihood of medication errors.

- Improved monitoring of people's health, preventing deterioration of LTCs and avoiding unnecessary healthcare usage.

This all supports the aims of the General Practice Forward View (GPFV 2016). TECS can help individuals live healthier lives, better manage their own health and well-being and reduce demand on local services so that the majority of the population can be supported in efficient ways, leaving traditional and increasingly scarce face-to-face resources focussed on those with complex conditions. TECS can also create vibrant patient communities enhancing collaboration amongst communities which in turn will help address problems associated with social isolation.

Case study: remote interactive patient and clinician consultations

In NHS Scotland, the 'Access Collaborative Programme' is a different way of bringing patients, clinicians and other NHS staff together to look at ways patients can receive timely and accessible care. A key focus is on ensuring patients won't be asked to travel unnecessarily and securing better access to specialists across the country through methods such as consultations with clinicians over secure virtual networks.

The programme has been developed to reduce planned waiting times by improving communications amongst staff working in the community and in hospitals to identify the right clinician and treatment and by streamlining patient care to minimise or eliminate unnecessary processes (Scottish Government 2016).

The key principles of the Access Collaborative Programme include the following:

- Patients shouldn't be asked to travel unless there is a clear clinical benefit, and any changes should increase the capacity and sustainability of the workload for primary, secondary and social care in a balanced way.
- All referrals should be either vetted by a consultant/senior decision maker or 'processed' via an agreed pathway or protocol.
- Referral and 'destination' pathways, including patient 'self-management' options, should be clear and published for all to see.
- Each hospital and referral system should have a joint and clear understanding of demand and capacity and how this matches with unscheduled care pathways and capacity.
- A clear understanding of access to diagnostics are part of pathway management.
- Improve metrics including how we record and measure virtual, telehealth, and tech-enabled care.

NHS Scotland has already been developing the use of virtual consultations through the Attend Anywhere platform whereby instead of travelling to their appointment, patients or service users enter the clinic's online waiting area from a web browser or app on their computers, smartphones, or tablets. The health service is notified when they arrive, and a provider joins the consultation when ready. Service users don't need to set up any kind of user account: they just click the 'Start video call' button on the health or care service's web page and follow the prompts (NHS Scotland 2018).

In addition to this, Florence telehealth system, a web-based clinical interface which collects data from patients via a mobile is also being used in the Western Isles of Scotland by the Western Isles Multiple Sclerosis service. They are using it to monitor patients' symptom management, medication compliance, exercise, weight and much more (Health Foundation 2018).

A PERSON-CENTRED APPROACH TO TECS

In essence person-centred care is simply the right care for the person's (or carer's) needs and preferences, delivered with dignity, compassion, sensitivity and respect, at the right time and place, with due regard to the person's age and any cognitive impairment. In addition, it includes the following:

- Holistic care that includes physical, mental, emotional, spiritual, social aspects and the person's own perspective and experiences – as appropriate.
- Shared care with informed, value based, preference sensitive, agreed between person (and carer/family if appropriate) and care professional.
- Safe care with informed decision making balancing potential benefits and risks where there are options for different routes and modes of delivery of care.
- Care designed with public and patient input and feedback.
- Proactive and inclusive of health promotion as well as primary, secondary and tertiary prevention.
- Methods integral to a quality improvement culture in health and social care.

All of these elements are relevant to the design and delivery of TECS in general practice – for individuals or groups of patients with the same LTC or those in need for behaviour change to redress their unhealthy lifestyle habits such as smoking or being too sedentary.

EXERCISE

So how can you enable a person (patient, carer or citizen) to participate in technology-enabled care to encourage them to take responsibility for their own health and wellbeing in your practice? Help them enhance their understanding and ownership of their LTC, lifestyle or frailty and enable them to engage in shared management with you and other care professionals and take more responsibility for their own health and wellbeing. So will you push them to take the following actions:

- Join in a telemedicine consultation with you for a review of their health condition.
- Use phone, text and instant messaging communications to receive information and reminders or interact with you.

- Signpost them to a mobile app related to their LTC or health and wellbeing to reinforce what you have advised or gain extra information about their treatment.
- Invite them to join a closed Facebook group that you or your practice has created that is relevant to their health condition or adverse lifestyle habit – then they will have peer-to-peer support as well as feedback from you or other member of the practice team.
- Encourage them to wear a monitoring device or other wearable technology for self-care such as a FitBit so they can bring or send you updates about their weight, blood pressure, and so on (as in Figure 5.1 at the lowest level).
- Refer them to assistive technology or telecare service related to their LTC, degree of frailty or health and wellbeing to enhance their safety and independence.

Being able to access their healthcare records remotely via the general practice computer system means that the patient can do the following:

- Review their own medical records.
- Order repeat prescription(s) online.
- Book a face-to-face appointment.
- Access the practice or other signposted health information website.
- Email requests to the general practice staff.

Those with an LTC or adverse lifestyle habit may then enhance their understanding of their condition(s) or state(s) and become more familiar with their treatments and associated test results. If deployed correctly, the patient will often dispense with the technology once it has taught them how to manage their condition. Thus they should be able to weigh the risks and benefits of potential treatment options offered and make intelligent choices. Then hopefully they will have greater adherence to treatment or interventions and set treatment goals related to clinical management of their LTC(s) or their adverse lifestyle habit(s). And this should result in prevention of deterioration of their LTC(s) or return to their adverse lifestyle habit(s) as a result of their active participation in technology-enabled care.

It might be thought axiomatic to develop and promote a person-centred approach to digital delivery of healthcare in general practice. To do that we need to accomplish the following:

- Understand what is really important to people about their health and care, taking into account their needs, preferences and personal circumstances.
- Empower citizens, patients and carers by making information about their health and wellbeing easily available.
- Encourage and support their access to, and use of, information about their health, including their health and social care records.

- Understand the limitations that exist within many practices both from an infrastructure and a skills perspective so as to tailor an approach that is deliverable and does not raise false expectations amongst patients.

Patients should be enabled (supported and educated) to gain the knowledge, skills and confidence they need to effectively manage their symptoms and condition(s) themselves so that they are able to make informed decisions and adhere to their medicines and treatment plans to achieve the best possible outcomes. A self-management plan or other care plan should be in an accessible format and include the following:

- Start and review dates.
- Descriptions of condition(s) or lifestyle habit(s) being managed.
- Current treatments including frequency of use, flexibility in doses of medicines and any restrictions.
- Arrangements for follow-up with a responsible care professional if the condition deteriorates, side effects from medicines and so on.

Digital solutions must be 'person centred'; based on the needs of the end user, whether that is a patient, carer, citizen or care professional. TECS are enablers, not an end in themselves.

WORKFORCE COMPETENCE AND CAPABILITY TO DEPLOY TECS

Primary care workforce teams should be supported to develop the skills and confidence needed to make effective use of digital modes of delivery or tools. These focus on the seven Cs relating to delivery of TECS (Chambers et al. 2018) for patients or citizens with LTCs or adverse lifestyle habits:

1 **Competence:** ability in relation to personal use of range of modes of delivery of TECS for agreed purpose, feeding information and acting on advice and information.
2 **Capability:** able to apply best practice in use of range of modes of delivery of TECS for agreed purpose, feeding information and acting on advice and information in daily professional and everyday life.
3 **Capacity:** possess protected and prioritised time for initiating and participating in remote delivery of care, which is regarded as key element of a nurse's work role – plus the IT infrastructure and equipment are available and easily accessed by all service providers and users.
4 **Confidence:** confident that organisational infrastructure is in place in line with the code of practice, including reliability and validity of equipment and its outputs, and confident that usage of TECS is integral part of clinical best practice and can access or act on relay of TECS messages or interchanges with patients.

5 **Creativity:** able to adopt and adapt agreed TECS for different purposes or patient and carer groups in line with the code of practice.
6 **Communication:** sharing and dissemination of digital modes of delivery and associated clinical protocols and evaluation of applications, outcomes, challenges and so on across the practice team, working together and sharing what has worked well and what has not worked so well.
7 **Continuity:** able to interact via mode of TECS along pathway(s) for LTCs or lifestyle habits, with cover arranged in the practice team as appropriate and pre-agreed with patients in line with agreed shared care management plans.

Promoting professional skills in person-centred digital care means focussing on the following:

Behavioural change

The National Institute for Health and Excellence (NICE) recommends a solution-focussed approach by care professionals that includes the following:

- Self-monitoring by patient or service user of behaviour and progress (with agreed shared care management plans and goals).
- Goal setting (mutually agreed by care professional and person [and carer]).
- Encouraging social support.
- Problem solving (with patient or service user encouraged to report issues).
- Encouraging patients and carers to be assertive.
- Cognitive restructuring by patient or carer (modifying thoughts).
- Reinforcement of changes (in behaviour, treatment, and interventions by the patient or carer).
- Relapse prevention and individualised strategies (NICE 2014).

Self-care, shared management

A shared management plan between patient and relevant care professionals should be a norm for a patient with an LTC or a person whose lifestyle habit may adversely affect his or her health. A clinician should be able to supply and engage people with appropriate decision aids (matching their values, preferences, knowledge and skills, ability, cognition, skills and motivation). The shared management plan should be agreed and accessible to all involved in delivery of care in line with patient informed consent.

Clinicians should aim to understand patients' perceptions of their health condition(s) and care to minimise barriers to their expected use of digital modes of delivery of care, giving them choice and control. They need a positive approach which focusses on what people who use their services can do or might be able to do with appropriate support, not what they cannot do.

Online access in general practice to a person's medical records, as well as booking of appointments and ordering repeat prescriptions, is increasingly available to patients. The rollout of online consultation platforms as part of the GP Forward View will make this even more accessible. Some patients can request that access to their general practice records is extended to other clinicians. So clinicians need to learn and understand appropriate clinical governance for safe-care management and information governance for conserving patient confidentiality and safe data sharing. Recent legislation has endorsed the use of a person's NHS number so that all organisations in health and social care identify the individual person in the same way with a view to sharing personal data in valid, reliable and safe ways.

NICE (2015) emphasises that putting people at the centre of decisions about their care can enable them to use prescribed medicines safely and effectively and get the best possible outcomes that the person values.

(iii) Shared decision making

Shared decision making is central to the delivery of evidence-based health or social care. Everyone should be offered the opportunity to be involved in making decisions about the delivery and scope of their care. Where there is more than one reasonable option, each with potential benefits and harms, the use of a high-quality patient decision aid can facilitate patient engagement and empower patient input into the choice of a selected option.

A patient decision aid should describe the options available in a way that the person is likely to understand and help the patient make an informed, value-based, preference-sensitive decision with the care professional after weighing the specific risks and benefits of options (NICE 2014).

IS YOUR ORGANISATION READY FOR PROVIDING TECS?

Adoption, rollout and development of any type of TECS delivery must adhere to all relevant quality and safety elements of a locally agreed code of practice which includes health and safety, information governance, clinical governance, indemnity, data sharing and security frameworks, assurance schemes and standards. An example code of practice agreed by the Staffordshire Digital Design Authority and thus endorsed by all health and social care organisations in Staffordshire is available on www.clinictecs.uk. It includes elements given as follows, collated from national standards set out by NHSE, the National Data Guardian, General Medical Council and other clinician regulatory councils.

Each general practice, as for any health and social care organisation, must agree to endorse and adhere to national requirements relating to IT security, clinical safety, data quality, the use of patient data, data protection and privacy and information standards. These include the following:

1 Information governance that defines standards and professional capability.
2 Clinical governance.

3 Legal and regulatory obligations and compliance with standards, for example, a privacy impact assessment and standard operating procedure endorsed by their Caldicott Guardian.
4 Procurement of technology and equipment such as medical devices.
5 Health and safety.
6 Quality management.
7 Care Quality Commission (CQC) requirements that include information security and governance.
8 NHSE requirements and priorities.
9 Identification of patient by NHS number.

In addition each practice should agree to endorse and adhere to good practice relating to the following:

- Upskilling staff (clinicians, managers and administrators) to establish competence and confidence in TECS within the organisation and networking with others in connected ways.
- Shared care management between clinicians and selected and signed-up patients, with synchrony amongst all organisations in the health economy for shared care management plans for all relevant care pathways and with delegated authority and responsibilities at organisational and individual patient levels.
- Valid, trustworthy, relevant and up-to-date data must be available when and where needed while also being accessible swiftly and securely for staff as well as within and amongst organisations.
- Explicit patient consent or opt-out option if or when it is proposed that patient personal confidential data is being used for purposes beyond direct care (unless there is a mandatory legal requirement or an overriding public interest in line with recent GDPR (Information Commissioners Office 2018).
- Patient safety reinforcing adherence to pre-agreed interventions between clinician and patient with underpinning delivery protocols focussed on specific selection criteria for patient groups.
- Clinical indemnity for practitioners delivering care via TECS instead of alternative modes of delivery of care.
- Security of transmission of care via TECS (e.g., Skype) underpinned by protocol describing patient selection criteria, setting, patient consent and so on.
- Measuring and demonstrating impact and collating evidence of positive outcomes and unintended consequences (safety risks and extra costs from additional workforce input).
- Contract management of performance.
- Monitoring and alerts.
- Reliable infrastructure for everyday relaying of TECS and associated equipment needed such as for bodily measurement by patients.
- Improve and sustain cybersecurity.
- Security standards for NHS mail in line with ISB 1596.

There should be formal risk management procedures in place in each practice to identify, report, document and investigate all incidents in relation to delivery of all types of clinical consultation. In parallel there should be a benefits analysis undertaken by the practice manager to oversee the effectiveness and productivity of the delivery of TECS to inform future implementation and aid sustainability. The practice provision of digital care should be in line with the five domains that the CQC has described as requirements for those providing healthcare by digital means. See the Table in Appendix 1 for extracts from the full CQC descriptors of the five domains (CQC 2017) that are relevant to the provision of TECS in general practice. They are, in the main, challenges from the CQC that the practice team needs to address proactively as they plan the set-up of digital delivery of care and then operate it with clinical oversight and/or non-clinical management.

CLINICAL CONSULTATION TYPES

Each clinician conducting a non-face-to-face consultation with a patient is responsible for ensuring that the mode and quality of the TECS for that consultation is of sufficient standard and scope for safe practice in relation to the patient's healthcare needs. If not, they should discontinue the consultation and arrange a different and more appropriate mode of clinical consultation to be delivered by themselves or other practitioner in a safe timescale.

Selecting a particular mode of consultation will depend on the need for shared decision making and shared management between patient and clinician; availability and accessibility of TECS (in relation to NHS and patient or carer ownership); patient's and carer's preference(s); self-care and/or continuity of care recommended; established relationship, trust and understanding between patient or carer and practitioner; whether follow-up or first presentation; severity and urgency of clinical management or prevention of disease or deterioration; availability of right type and level of clinician; appropriate risk management; working across organisational boundaries; making the best use of technology; whether the mode of TECS is affordable and sustainable; quality, safety and efficiency; expected outcomes being clear and reasonable; the existence of good quality and safety underpinning the mode of TECS; the competence and confidence of practitioner(s) involved; and patient and carer to use preferred mode(s) of TECS.

It is the responsibility of each clinician to select patients for an appropriate mode of consultation depending on their symptoms, signs, cognition, support, confidence and preferences. This might be face-to-face or any mode of digital delivery of care. Selection criteria should be modified to take account of clinicians' experience and specialty as well as accessibility and availability of TECS and the patients' needs and preferences. Face-to-face consultation differs from remote modes of consultation such as telephone or email interactions as the clinician assessment includes the patient's (and carer's) body language and non-verbal communication, such as facial expressions, as well as the opportunity to undertake physical examination.

Innovative consultation modes, where technology is a given component include telephone consultations (Pygall 2017), email or online consultations and video consultations. A full analysis is beyond the scope of this chapter, and for the most part they are at an early stage of development. Nonetheless it is almost inevitable that these forms of non-traditional clinician and patient interaction will expand over the next few years. Group interactions are being currently researched, a variant of which are interactions via social media, also in their infancy.

EXERCISE

Plan your own adoption of technology-enabled care in your practice:

1 What is the problem or issue for which you might focus a mode of digital delivery of care? Is that connected to the delivery of LTC care or redressing of an adverse lifestyle habit?

- *Which problem or issue will you address?*
- *Who will your planned delivery of digital care involve or affect?*

2 Define the baseline measurement and evaluation.

- *Before you start how will you measure or assess the scale and scope of the problem? Will you or others in your practice team collect baseline data?*
- *What will you measure, and how will you or others measure it?*

3 Describe your plan for providing digital delivery of care in your practice.

- *What will you do?*
- *How will you engage with others in the practice and patients in identifying the problems or issues and designing the solution?*
- *When will the intervention start (date), and over what period will it run?*

And then record your results and findings

4 What were the findings?

- *What were your end-of-project results (exactly what did you measure and how did you measure it – have you collated any tables or figures)?*

5 Describe patient and stakeholder engagement.

What engagement did you undertake with patients/practice team members and others, for example, CCG in the following:

- *Identifying the problem.*
- *Designing the intervention.*
- *Understanding or interpreting the findings.*
- *Planning follow up actions.*

6 Look backwards and forwards.

- *What feedback – positive and negative – did you get, for example, from patients and carers, practice staff and commissioners?*

- *What challenges did you face? Did you overcome them? How?*
- *If you repeated the project, what would you do differently?*
- *Has your intervention now become routine practice? If yes, will it be sustainable in the long term? If no, why not?*

7   Give brief overall costs; for example, include staff salaries, equipment and facilities.

CONCLUSIONS

It is inevitable that primary care will need to adapt to the relentless march of technology in the same way that other aspects of daily life have needed to in recent years (Castle-Clark and Imison 2016). In doing so the role of the regulators is beginning to be felt increasingly (Coleman 1997) evident, and it is likely that their role will increase over time. We have described the potential for the improvement in patient care that TECS may bring, acknowledging that day-to-day changes in the delivery of primary care will be necessary. The scope for evaluation of such changes is to be hoped for as a counterweight to changes brought about simply by the pressure of events.

REFERENCES

Care Quality Commission (2017) Clarification of regulatory methodology: PMS digital healthcare providers. www.cqc.org.uk/sites/default/files/20170303_pms-digital-healthcare_regulatory-guidance.pdf

Castle-Clarke, S. and Imison, C. (2016) *The digital patient: Transforming primary care.* London: Nuffield Trust. https://www.nuffieldtrust.org.uk/research/the-digital-patient-transforming-primary-care

Chambers, R., Schmid, M., Al Jabbouri, A. and Beanery, P. (2018) *Making digital healthcare happen in practice: A practical handbook.* Oxford: Otmoor Publishing.

Chambers, R., Schmid, M. and Birch-Jones, J. (2016) *Digital healthcare: The essential guide.* Oxford: Otmoor Publishing. https://itun.es/gb/k_Xveb.l

Coleman, A. (1997) Where do I stand? Legal implications of telephone triage. *Journal of Clinical Nursing,* 6(3): 227–231.

Health Foundation (2018) www.health.org.uk/content/overview-florence-simple-telehealth-text-messaging-system-flo (accessed 13.5.19)

Information Commissioner's Office (2018) https://ico.org.uk/for-organisations/guide-to-the-general-data-protection-regulation-gdpr/ (accessed 13.5.19)

NHS England (2016) *General practice forward view.* NHS England, Leeds. www.england.nhs.uk/wp-content/uploads/2016/04/gpfv.pdf (accessed 13.5.19)

NHS Scotland (2018) *Attend anywhere.* https://sctt.org.uk/programmes/video-enabled-health-and-care/attendanywhere/ (accessed 13.5.19)

NICE (2014) *Obesity: Identification, assessment and management.* www.nice.org.uk/guidance/cg189

NICE (2015) *Medicines optimisation: The safe and effective use of medicines to enable the best possible outcomes.* NICE Guideline 5. www.nice.org.uk/guidance/ng5

Pygall, S.A. (2017) *Telephone triage and consultation.* London: RCGP.

Scottish Government (2016) *The modern outpatient: A collaborative approach 2017–2020.* https://news.gov.scot/news/reducing-planned-waiting-times (accessed 13.5.19)

CQC domains for digital healthcare

....

Five domains that the CQC require of providers of digital healthcare		
CQC domain	**TECS elements in place?**	**Yes/No – details?**
Safe?	Is there a clinical protocol in place? Is there specific individualised advice for different patient groups as opposed to generic advice? Is personal data held? Can it be viewed? Can the participating patient's identity be seen by anyone who should not have sight of it?	
Effective?	What happens if a participating patient needs a face-to-face consultation after remote interaction? Have a participant's needs been established in the set-up of the technology?	
Caring?	Has participant consent been obtained? How? Has a privacy impact assessment been undertaken? Has the participating patient been advised how to protect online information?	
Responsive?	Does the participating patient understand the limitations of the remote care service? Is the patient's access limited by space or time? How accessible is the selected mode(s) of delivery of TECS?	
Well led?	How does the provider ensure oversight by manager and/or clinician of TECS? How does the provider ensure the TECS offer is person centred?	
Take a look at the full guidance – www.cqc.org.uk/sites/default/files/20170303_pms-digital-healthcare_regulatory-guidance.pdf		

CHAPTER 6

Collaboration in general practice

....

Jo Sauvage

LEARNING OBJECTIVES

- Explain why collaboration in general practice is fundamental to the provision of optimal patient care in GP.
- Determine why collaboration is fundamental to the way we transform services to achieve the 'holy grail' of sustainability.
- Describe why this is especially important now.
- Outline how patient care is being improved through different forms of collaboration.
- Explain how this is influencing the role of the GP within the delivery of future healthcare in England.

THE MEANING OF COLLABORATION

Collaboration is the act of working together with other people or organisations to create or achieve something (Cambridge University Press 2018). Over my career as a GP I have refined how I can best collaborate with my patients, other professionals and services so that patients get the care they need and my daily practice remains productive. During this time, I have witnessed the scope and the need for collaboration to change (Baird et al. 2018; Baird 2018).

Synonyms for 'collaboration' include words such as 'partnership', cooperation' and 'alliance', and despite the fact that GPs to date have remained independent contractors within the NHS hierarchy, all these descriptors have at some point been aligned with the word 'GP'. The descriptors also track the adaptations the profession has made over time, as it continues to evolve from the historical image of single-handed practitioner working from residential premises, through several metamorphoses, to meet changing patient needs and growing demand (Baird et al. 2018; Baird 2018). Paradoxically, the word 'collaboration' has been less ascribed historically to general practice but is the most apt now as we seek to find new solutions to respond to the growing pressures facing our profession, both in England (Baird et al. 2016) and internationally (Rosen 2013).

REASONS FOR GPS TO BE PART OF A TEAM

Core to general practice has always been the delivery of family medicine to people of all ages, from a community-based setting, at the heart of which is continuity of care and patient advocacy (Gilbert 2013). Growing population need is driving the move to provide care from a more cost-effective setting. All health economies continue to look for ways to make healthcare sustainable, and the increasing repatriation of care to GPs is a consequence of this. Thus, over the past twenty years the complexity of care delivered within general practice has increased exponentially (Baird et al. 2016). General practice has already responded over this time by varying the skills of employed staff, such that team-based care is the established norm. However, whilst collaboration amongst professionals in primary care and across organisational interfaces has always been key to excellence in clinical care, this now needs to go one step further.

Significant pressures in recruitment and retention of GPs and practice nurses, coupled with reduced resources, have negatively affected workload and the capacity to deliver high-quality services from all practices. GP morale is low (Gilbert 2013; Healthy London Partnership 2018), and practices are at increased risk of closure as the resilience of the traditional small business model is fragile. These are some of the reasons contributing to variation in access to appointments, the range of services provided to patients as well as variation in patient outcomes.

In addition to these issues, pay-for-performance strategies adopted in general practice have provided an inaccurate view of general practice alone and its place within a larger system (Roland et al. 2016). The ethos of what is important in care delivery has matured, and although we recognise the importance of using data to drive quality, we need a more sophisticated framework, able to capture, for example, the management of complexity as well as a more person-centred offer to patient's dependent on their needs and which requires collaboration with others to achieve the best outcomes (Roland et al. 2016; Baird et al. 2018).

In response to the changing landscape and an attempt to describe the need for an adaptable service requirement, some areas have started to re-define the response descriptors from general practice; for example, in London's 'Transforming Primary Care', new core elements were stated as the provision of accessible, pro-active and co-ordinated care (NHS England 2015). This drives the definition of quality to also be about timely access to appointments; it acknowledges the importance of preventative interventions and the need for care to be organised and easy to navigate. It is the modern translation of what was articulated in 1992 by Barbara Starfield as the four pillars of primary care practice: first-contact care, continuity of care, comprehensive care and coordination of care (Starfield 1994).

Further to this, the Forward View for GPs (NHSE et al. 2016) has defined the need for general practice to transform its current model to be better able to respond to the needs of the population as it evolves over the next twenty years. This includes a vision for a changing workforce, ways of working and the scope of the job. This narrative of system transformation signals the need for greater collaboration amongst general practices, reaching out across organisational interfaces and greater functional integration across health and social care, physical and mental health, primary care and acute services, working together around the needs of a population (Baird et al. 2018).

In *Next Steps to the Strategic Commissioning Framework – A Vision for Strengthening General Practice Collaboration across London* (Healthy London Partnership 2018), the idea of general practices specifically working collaboratively together is further developed, with large-scale general practices working together through a variety of different models to optimise care for patients in their geographical area. This is commonplace across England with the aim of working together to strengthen resilience, reduce variation, support and maintain our clinical workforce and strengthen administrative processes, for example, by the merger of back office functions and application of consistent processes. The NHS Long-Term Plan (NHS 2019) defines the role of general practice in the next phase of this transformation into integrated care systems (NHS 2019) with GP services working at scale providing a bridge not only horizontally with other practices but also vertically into specialist services within hospital-based care and mental health organisations.

The evolving clinical and social complexity of the GP caseload means that we can no longer work in isolation. Pathways of care require a team-based and collaborative approach, with sub-optimal patient care delivered where this does not work well. This is the essence of the themes highlighted in the National Voices, 'I statements', for delivering better person-centred care, at the heart of which are processes and enablers that systematically support collaboration amongst professionals and with their patients and service users (Department of Health & Social Care 2013). The practical manifestations of these enablers include integrated IT to support easier information sharing, multi-disciplinary meetings and most importantly interpersonal relationships and effective team culture at all organisational levels to drive this (West 2013) – in short, better integration of services around patient's needs with general practice at the core.

EXERCISE

- How much do you know about the organisation of GP services in your local area?
- Why is this important, and how can you find out more?

THE NATURE OF COLLABORATION TODAY AND TOMORROW

Professional roles and clinical care

As the nature of the work in general practice has changed, so the nature of the workforce supporting its delivery has significantly evolved. The practice team is now fashioned by the need to collaborate across a wide range of people and professions. This is, in part, due to the need to diversify skill mix so that care is delivered by the person with the right skills the first time, in part due to the need to bolster capacity and capability through the development and emergence of new roles. New roles include GP assistants, care navigators, physician associates and advanced care practitioners (Baird et al. 2018), not forgetting the increasing secondary care medical workforce who are working in primary and community care to support the management of complexity with advanced specialist skills. It will take time to be able to fully realise the potential of this new capability and capacity within the system (Baird 2018).

Practice-based pharmacists can optimise prescribing so that it is safe, evidence-based and provides value as well as providing support for LTC management (Shah et al. 2015; NHSE et al. 2016). Healthcare assistants support the work of GPs and practice nurses in monitoring and disease-prevention strategies; community specialist nurses provide specific and intensive support for LTCs such as chronic obstructive pulmonary disease (COPD) or heart failure; and community matrons provide generalist case management for patients at high risk of admission to hospital, helping keep people at home.

Management advice and guidance from specialists to GPs and other community partners can be given via email in real time to avoid unnecessary visits to hospital or waits for outpatient appointments. More urgent assessment with access to diagnostic tests and specialist assessment can be achieved without the need for admission due to better collaboration amongst the hospital and primary care clinicians along 'ambulatory care pathways'; patients are seen in a 'one-stop shop' for diagnostic tests and treatment, reducing the need to be admitted to hospital and improving the patient experience (Barker et al. 2017).

Case study: collaboration to improve quality, efficiency and safety

City Road Medical Centre is an inner London practice and has had problems with recruitment and retention of GPs and practice nurses. The practice was included as a case study in a review to understand the undocumented pressures in GPs (Baird 2016). To overcome the recruitment problems, the partners decided to recruit a practice-based pharmacist. Working closely with the pharmacist and with a dedicated administrator, they streamlined the management of repeat prescribing and medication reviews. Each GP saved more than forty-five minutes every day, whereas the patients were more satisfied with the service and there were fewer prescribing errors.

When a patient is discharged from hospital, the discharge team talks to the pharmacist to make sure that the prescription is updated and the appropriate medication ready for when the person gets home. Each week the practice holds a multi-disciplinary meeting, during which any patients of concern can be discussed. These are patients at risk of admission or those soon to be discharged so that the combined resources of the wider team collaborate, drawing on each other's skills and expertise to achieve the best outcomes for the patient. Multi-disciplinary members attend, including matrons who work across the hospital – community interface thus bridging the transition.

In recognition of the importance of well-being, a navigator works with patients to understand what is most important to them then draws on collaboration from voluntary sector organisations to provide support that is 'more than medicine', such as befriending services or other activities to combat social isolation.

Interventions such as this have developed a sense of collective understanding, teamwork, improved staff and patient experience and reduced length of stay and readmission rates (Nesta 2011).

Multi-disciplinary teams and networks

As the number of people involved in the management of a case can now be significant, this requires not only collaboration but coordination: collaboration, so that the individual patients and their teams work to the best effect together to achieve the best outcomes, and coordination, as for patients with complex needs, it is important that the professionals are brought together most effectively to collaborate. This is the domain of the multi-disciplinary team meeting (MDT), either face-to-face or virtual; the needs of a complex person can be discussed, and an appropriate management plan made and then monitored. Organisational infrastructure and administrative support are required to undertake the practical requirements of meeting coordination.

The clinical co-ordinator is the named person who links the person's needs and goals to what care is delivered and how. The GP can be optimally placed to act as the clinical co-ordinator, bringing continuity of care and an understanding of the holistic needs and goals of the patient to support the delivery of the best outcomes. Indeed, evidence suggests that this continuity of care can reduce unnecessary hospital admissions and provides better patient experience (Jeffers et al. 2016). However, commensurate with patient need, co-ordination to support collaboration can also be achieved by other professional groups; non-clinical navigators are important and able to signpost or actively support patients to utilise the widest range of services, including alternative pathways. Such may rely on a more holistic approach, such as social prescribing, which helps mobilise personal assets and capacity to better self-manage and is a way of linking patients in primary care with valuable sources of support within the community (Gilburt et al. 2018).

This wider collaboration of multi-disciplinary professionals is also about tangibly and visibly working together in a given place – a locality or neighbourhood – a place that people would recognise as where they live and where they go regularly. This is now described as an 'integrated network' delivering place-based care. This is about how services are organised so that they are visible and understood by the people using them and, where possible, are delivered locally. The intention to address a person's holistic needs is implicit, working in partnership with local communities, voluntary sector organisations and with links into the local authority to enable the wider determinants of disease and wellbeing to be addressed, such as public health, housing and employment. It includes primary and secondary care and mental health provision as well. Future design will create the widest offer of integrated local services wrapped around the heart of general practice, hence the need to extend the opportunities and systems to enable the widest collaboration for the benefit of patients as well as welcoming the involvement of volunteers (Gilburt et al. 2018).

Supporting mechanisms and processes

Although a person's health and care needs may require different components of support to be provided by different organisations, all they want to experience is a system that works for them and is easy to navigate; the same must be said for workers. Why make the job difficult? Thus, how the system functions is paramount and trumps any attempts to standardise its organisational form. To deliver improved function with better quality, safer services and positive user experience, we must actively work to ensure that collaboration across boundaries exists. Methods that build and maintain relationships are fundamental to this as these are the foundations from which the energy for change and joy in working are rooted (National Improvement & Leadership Development Board 2018).

To facilitate greater collaboration across professions, we need to better understand each other's roles and scopes of practice. It is also important to understand the differences at each end of a pathway of care – from specialist hospital to GP surgery and out into the person's home. The delivery of education in a way that is collaborative, multi-disciplinary and grounded in a place plants the seeds of success for future collaborative work as people work together and learn together. The Community Education Provider Networks (CEPNs) are founded on this principle (Healthy London Partnership 2016).

To work together in a coordinated and integrated way to share in the responsibility of delivering care, staff must be able to communicate and share information and know where the accountability for care sits. This is complex in a community environment where members of the team may all be working for different organisations. However, in terms of delivering the best outcomes for patients, it is vital that staff collectively make every contact count (National Institute for Health & Care Guidance 2007, 2011) and have the governance to do this. Through working in this way and collaborating across organisations, it becomes possible for all partners to share information such as disease registers and then take collective responsibility to manage the outcomes of patients in their area. Through collaborating on data sharing, comparing outcomes and working together to address variation through the systematic use of quality improvement methodology, significant improvements in population healthcare can be achieved (Royal College of GPs 2018). It is however important to ensure that clear governance processes are established and understood so as not to hinder the safe delivery of a transformed model of care. This is especially important regarding data management both for delivering individual care as well as the utilisation of disease registers and predictive analytics.

Organisational collaboration to standardise staff terms and conditions or remuneration amongst employing organisations including general practice can help reduce staff turnover exacerbated by organisations competing for staff. Collaboration to develop innovative posts and 'blended roles' working across primary and secondary care can attract and retain staff as well as providing portfolio careers with opportunities for professional development. Such opportunities encourage recruitment and retention and bring the benefits of a stable workforce, as well as the practical understanding of how to manage a patient across a whole pathway of care, which carries future benefits.

Knowledge, skills and attitudes

The core competencies of the UK RCGP curriculum for specialist training include competency domains such as 'optimising communication skills', 'data gathering and interpretation', and 'managing medical complexity', which are essential to the safe and effective management of undifferentiated clinical problems within the context of the consultation. The growing background complexity within the GP environment make less clinically oriented competencies just as essential to providing good care and support the drive towards working collaboratively; these domains include 'working with colleagues and in teams', 'community orientation' and, recently added, 'organisation, management and leadership (Royal College of GPs 2016).

Attitude is an important ingredient of working in collaboration at every level as it fundamentally requires a shift towards a universally non-hierarchical approach in which all team members are respected for providing a valid, important element of care. Whilst there has been a growing move towards values-based recruitment (away from the historical approach largely dependent on skills and experience), a new methodology to deliver workforce education and development is required to foster this non-hierarchical approach as the status quo within multi-disciplinary teams. There are well-documented examples of how historical preconceptions of professions act as a legacy to pre-determine behaviours and attitudes which can influence the delivery of patient care. This is described for the social worker–doctor relationship (RCGP et al. 2014) but equally exists amongst the professionals working across different disciplines: physical, mental health or primary and secondary care.

CEPNs have been developed in some areas as the platform to support collaborative multi-disciplinary education. The network is the fulcrum that enables front-line workers to drive the delivery of educational initiatives that they need to support what they do. It is developed by and delivered to an integrated workforce and not in disciplinary silos (Healthy London Partnership 2016).

It is this culture change in the way education is delivered that will drive a more egalitarian and naturally collaborative approach in the way people work together to provide better patient care. This integrated way of providing education and development is being recognised as vitally important at postgraduate and undergraduate levels, with the development of new and innovative curricula for the latter (Kent & Medway Medical School 2018).

Patient engagement and patient participation

Working in collaboration with patients and carers has always been fundamental to support shared decision making. Postgraduate education for GPs universally includes some reflection on consultation models as one of the fundamental enablers to better understand how to communicate effectively. We now recognise the importance of 'collaboration' as a skill set, important to both sides of the partnership. Patient empowerment or 'activation' results from having the knowledge and skills to collaborate actively in the consultation and subsequently in the delivery of self-care.

It can be taught to both service users and deliverers of care and used to enhance motivation and confidence in self-management when linked to the achievement of goals that are important to the individual. It is the bilateral collaboration between the doctor and patient that creates success, supported by the collaboration of systems and processes that make this way of working possible. This is the basis of the House of Care model of delivering improvements in LTC management through supporting positive behaviour change (Year of Care Partnerships 2011; Sauvage et al. 2016; Chambers et al. 2016).

Finally, it is collaboration with residents and patients through formal engagement, in practices via patient participation groups, or on a larger scale at the level of CCGs that is strategically important. It is a statutory requirement of both organisations and facilitates the co-design, development and commissioning of services that people want and need. This commissioning cycle is the way that services are planned, developed and monitored, paid for and improved (from GP practices to the wider system), and the link with residents and users is a key element in this process.

EXERCISE

- What experience have you had observing or participating in collaborative work to improve patient care?
- What have you identified to be the important factors?
- Can you identify areas in which improved collaboration could bring about real benefits for patients, staff, and ways of working?
- What steps could be taken to do this?

LEADERSHIP FOR EFFECTIVE COLLABORATION AND EVOLUTION

Effective collaboration requires leadership and willingness to manage one's own work effectively but also help the organisation and others respond and adapt. Within the clinical domain of day-to-day practice, GPs will take a leadership role in the coordination of duties for that session of work, collaborating with all other team members to manage demand and clinical needs effectively and safely. In the context of the traditional small business model of GP practice management, partners work in collaboration with the practice manager and senior administrators to manage the business side, which includes finances, human resources, estates management and patient liaison. Whilst there are benefits derived from this established small-scale business model, many disadvantages prevail, including unnecessary duplication, wasted resource due to the associated opportunity cost and reduced resilience by delivering services at reduced scale. In addition, due to problems with recruitment and retention of staff, the cost of agency staff and the expanding nature of the role of GP, capacity must be directed to front-line patient care with less time available for formal management, organisational development or quality improvement. The delivery of quality care is best done by supporting GPs and clinical leaders to obtain education and training in quality improvement methods and developing organisational cultures where leaders and staff focus on better value as a primary goal. Not creating the time for this is to the detriment of quality care as these areas are vital to the successful running of the organisation and service delivery (Ham et al. 2016; National Improvement & Leadership Development Board 2018).

Within a practice, GP leadership is vital in supporting initiatives which improve productivity and release more time for patient care. The RCGP has made recommendations on how this might be achieved. In 'Spotlight on the 10 High Impact Actions' (RCGP 2018), many of the actions advocated are delivered through greater collaboration at multiple levels, for example, productive workflows being best achieved through greater collaboration between clinicians and practice staff. Administrative staff can develop advanced skills to safely stream patients or signpost them into alternative, more appropriate services as well as support the management of other clinical duties, such as timely summarising and streamlining of clinical mail and managing referrals and administrative enquiries from external sources. Some general practices have responded to resilience challenges by list expansion, with larger lists often able to provide greater revenue stability, staffing numbers as well as a wider range of services.

However, many GPs are not able to manage the balance of clinical care delivery and practice management whilst maintaining an eye for this evolutionary change. This is even more poignant the smaller the scale for operational delivery. A recognised way to universally support practices to drive greater productivity and provide greater resilience is the opportunity offered by working at scale in federated or networked models. GP practices collaborate to participate in service delivery, share registers to manage specific cohorts of patients or share infrastructure, such as back office functions or staff. There are national models that achieve this; what is important is helping local practices come together to implement this new way of working. It is only GPs who can lead peer colleagues to do this – to make collaboration on a broader scale standard practice, systematically undertaken at multiple levels across organisations. GP leadership is required to help reconcile in the minds of colleagues the virtues of traditional practice with the opportunities inherent in the transformational vision for general practice of the future. GP leadership is essential to help peers understand the need for transformation as well as how to do this.

Without the opportunity of time for strategic thinking, none of the innovation will ever take place (Baird 2018). Given the financial constraints that exist and the opportunity cost of taking people out of clinical practice to implement change, it will be difficult to make the transformational vision real unless there is collaboration. Capacity for change can only be realised where service delivery is provided with some economy of scale and people work together to deliver the vision.

GP leadership is a vital ingredient to successful collaboration to improve health and care delivery for patients and residents through bringing to bare the intimate knowledge of patient experience of illness and health as well as the impact of existing services on health improvement and disease prevention. In their capacity as clinical leaders within the commissioning of services, GPs in CCGs have collaborated with local authority colleagues and providers of services to strive to ensure that populations receive the services that they need. It has been collaboration at this strategic level, across partner organisations and public-sector partners, that has resulted in the optimisation of clinical pathways to deliver better patient outcomes.

The Better Care Fund was established in 2013 as the programme vehicle spanning both the NHS and local government and providing the opportunity for unique collaboration amongst NHS England, the Department of Health and Social Care (DHSC), the local government and housing. The four partners work closely together to help local areas plan and implement integrated health and social care services across England in line with the vision outlined in the NHS FYFV.

It was created to improve the lives of some of the most vulnerable people in society, placing them at the centre of their care and support and providing them integrated health and social care services, resulting in an improved experience and better quality of life.

There are many examples in which such system leadership and financial collaboration have brought about improvements at the patient level. For example, in April 2016 Greater Manchester took charge of the £6 billion spent on health and social care through a devolution deal with the government. The region also received an extra resource to support transformation which brought together local organisations, including local councils and the NHS CCGs, to create the Greater Manchester Health and Social Care Partnership.

The partnership has implemented a huge range of new initiatives to improve the health and wellbeing of its population. For example, Wigan's community nurses work alongside social care staff and therapists to support people with LTCs at home, whereas in Bolton a new service is helping people with chaotic lifestyles. Both initiatives mean people need hospital treatment less frequently (NAPC 2018).

The success of GP collaboration at senior leadership level has however had a limited impact to date in driving sustainable transformation in the delivery of care in England. This limited success is more related to the impact of the Health and Care Act 2011 on the NHS landscape than the lack of collaborative intent from GP leadership and other system partners to achieve it. The act produced a system designed to respond to an historical set of problems and an ideology that improvements in care could be achieved through greater competition, manifest through use of market tendering and activity-based payments rather than collaboration between providers and integration of services. The next phase of transition for the English NHS is set to circumvent this through the evolution of integrated care systems, where the focus of operation will be to achieve greater alignment and collaboration at both clinical and organisational levels, with a significant reduction in transaction cost, to go in part to support longer-term value and sustainability.

Whatever definitive form is achieved, the centre of gravity for collaboration, coordination and system leadership must reside as close to the patient and primary care practitioners as possible to achieve this.

EXERCISE

- Are there any areas of learning you can identify that will improve the care you provide patients individually or in the context of the wider system within which you operate (i.e., quality improvement methodology or leadership skills)?
- What steps will help you achieve these goals, and how will you know you have achieved them?

GPS AND WIDER SYSTEM COLLABORATION

Due to the progression of advances in medical science, we are now able to do so much more. We are struggling through this phase of evolution at this moment because of the universal desire to deliver equitable services to a growing population with increased need and expectations in circumstances of financial austerity. Constraints on the supply of resources can devastate the outputs of carefully nurtured collaborations based on relationships and trust. This is as true in the context of the GP consultation with, for example, restricted treatments, as in that of organisational collaboration and the management of financial risk.

It is the fundamental collaboration between the GP and the patient that is important in bringing to light the reality of what a person and his or her community needs and translating this into service design and delivery through subsequent collaborations both horizontally within teams and vertically to inform strategy. Ultimately, a strong, jointly owned vision of a better future needs to be co-developed and owned by all partners, including patients, to cement collaborative intent as the modus operandi and not allow the need for NHS transformation to be thwarted by the complexity of the task.

CONCLUSION

Whilst this narrative has been written at a point in time when there exists a crescendo sense of urgency to manage population health and population need in a way that is equitable and sustainable, this has been an eternal conundrum in the NHS and is mirrored in other health economies, irrespective of supporting payment mechanisms. I have described how improving both status quo and system transformation depends on collaboration and new ways of collaboration between people and organisations.

At present despite some areas of advanced development, systems work in a locally driven, variable and inconsistent manner, giving rise to unwarranted variation in the quality of care a person receives. It has proved difficult to date to seek to achieve a systematic approach within many health systems. Whilst this may be driven by many variables, the need for collaboration and positive working relationships is a universal and omnipresent truth in the effective delivery of health and care services.

Understanding the importance of collaboration in general practice is therefore vital to professional training, given the key role of the GP to the future model of delivery of care.

REFERENCES

Baird, B. (September 2018) *Blog: Shaping the future of general practice*, Kings Fund Publications. https://www.kingsfund.org.uk/blog/2018/09/shaping-future-general-practice. Accessed 30th May 2019.

Baird, B. et al. (2016) *Understanding pressures in general practice*, Kings Fund Publications. https://www.kingsfund.org.uk/sites/default/files/field/field_publication_file/Understanding GP-pressures-Kings-Fund-May-2016.pdf. Accessed 30th May 2019.

Baird, B. et al. (June 2018) *Innovative models of GP*, Kings Fund Publications. https://www.kingsfund.org.uk/sites/default/files/2018-06/Innovative_models_GP_summary_Kings_Fund_June_2018.pdf. Accessed 30th May 2019.

Barker, et al. (2017) Association between continuity of care in general practice and hospital admissions for ambulatory care sensitive conditions: Cross sectional study of routinely collected, person level data *BMJ*, 356: j84.

Cambridge Dictionary. Cambridge University Press (2018). https://dictionary.cambridge.org/dictionary/english/. Accessed 30th May 2019.

Chambers, E. and Coleman, K. (2016) Enablers and barriers for engaged, informed individuals and carers: Left wall of the House of Care framework. *British Journal of General Practice*. doi:10.3399/bjgp16X683797.

Department of Health and Social Care (May 2013) *Integrated care: Our shared commitment*. A framework that outlines ways to improve health and social care integration. https://assets.publishing.service.gov.uk/government/uploads/system/uploads/attachment_data/file/198748/DEFINITIVE_FINAL_VERSION_Integrated_Care_and_Support_-_Our_Shared_Commitment_2013-05-13.pdf. Accessed 30th May 2019.

Gilbert, J. (November 2013) *Transforming primary care in London: General practice: A call to action*, NHS England (London Region).

Gilburt, H. et al. (February 2018) *Volunteering in general practice Opportunities and insights*, Kings Fund Publications. https://www.kingsfund.org.uk/sites/default/files/2018-02/Volunteering-in-general-practice-full-report.pdf. Accessed 30th May 2019.

Ham, C. et al. (February 2016) *Improving quality in the English NHS: A strategy for action*, Kings Fund Publications. https://www.kingsfund.org.uk/sites/default/files/field/field_publication_file/Improving-quality-Kings-Fund-February-2016.pdf. Accessed 30th May 2019.

Health London Partnership (March 2016) *Community Education Provider Networks (CEPNs)*. London and the South East. https://www.healthylondon.org/wp-content/uploads/2017/11/CEPNs-in-London-and-the-South-East.pdf. Accessed 30th May 2019.

Healthy London Partnership (2018) *The next steps to the strategic commissioning framework: A vision for strengthening general practice collaboration across London*. www.healthy london.org/resource/the-next-steps-to-the-strategic-commissioning-framework/. Accessed 2018.

Jeffers, H. et al. (2016) *Continuity of care in modern day general practice*, Royal College of General Practitioners. https://bjgp.org/content/66/649/396. Accessed May 2019.

Kent and Medway Medical School (2018) Online prospectus. https://kmms.canterbury.ac.uk/kent-and-medway-medical-school.aspx. Accessed 2018.

NAPC (November 2018) *Primary care home and social care: Working together*. www.napc.co.uk. Accessed 2018.

National Improvement and Leadership Development Board Update (August 2018) *Developing people: Improving care: A national framework for action on improvement and leadership development in NHS-funded services*. https://improvement.nhs.uk/documents/542/Developing_People-Improving_Care-010216.pdf. Accessed 30th May 2019.

National Institute for Health & Care Guidance (October 2007) *Public Health Guideline (PH6) behaviour change: General approaches*. https://www.nice.org.uk/guidance/ph6/resources/behaviour-change-general-approaches-pdf-55457515717. Accessed May 30th 2019.

National Institute for Health & Care Guidance (December 2011) *Making every contact count: Implementing* NICE behaviour change guidance https://www.nice.org.uk/sharedlearning/making-every-contact-count-implementing-nice-behaviour-change-guidance. Accessed May 30th 2019.

Nesta (2011) *People powered health*. www.nesta.org.uk/project/people-powered-health/. Accessed 2018.

NHS (January 2019) *The NHS long term plan*. www.longtermplan.nhs.uk. Accessed 2019.

NHS England (2015) *Transforming primary care in London: A strategic commissioning framework*. www.england.nhs.uk/london/wp-content/uploads/sites/8/2015/03/lndn-prim-care-doc.pdf. Accessed 2018.

NHSE, RCGP and NHS HEE (April 2016) *GP forward view policy statement gateway 05116*. https://www.england.nhs.uk/wp-content/uploads/2016/04/gpfv.pdf. Accessed 30th May 2019.

RCGP and The College of Social work (October 2014) *GPs and social workers: Partners for better care delivering health and social care integration together*. A report by The College of Social Work and the Royal College of General Practitioners www.basw.co.uk/system/files/resources/basw_104434-7_0.pdf. Accessed 2018.

Roland, M. et al. (2016) Quality and outcomes framework: What have we learnt? *BMJ*, 354: i4060.

Rosen, R. (12 December 2013) Common challenges, common solutions: Lessons from primary care in Europe. *Nuffield Trust Comment*. www.nuffieldtrust.org.uk/news-item/common-challenges-common-solutions-lessons-from-primary-care-in-europe. Accessed 2018.

Royal College of General Practitioners (January 2016) *The RCGP curriculum: Professional & clinical modules 2.01–3.21 curriculum modules*. https://www.gmc-uk.org/-/media/documents/RCGP_Curriculum_modules_jan2016.pdf_68839814.pdf. Accessed 30th May 2019.

Royal College of General Practitioners (May 2018) *Spotlight on the 10 high impact actions*. https://www.rcgp.org.uk/policy/general-practice-forward-view/spotlight-on-the-10-high-impact-actions.aspx.

Sauvage, J. and Ahluwalia, S. (2016) Health and care professionals committed to partnership working: Right wall of the house of care framework. *British Journal of General Practice.* doi:10.3399/bjgp16X683389.

Shah, R. et al. (April 2015) *The benefits of working with an in-practice pharmacist.* www.gponline.com/benefits-working-in-practice-pharmacist/article/1341201. Accessed 2018.

Starfield, B. (October 1994) Is primary care essential? *The Lancet,* 344(8930): 1129–1133.

West, M. (February 2013) *Developing cultures of high quality care,* Kings Fund Publications. www.kingsfund.org.uk/sites/default/files/michael-west-developing-cultures-%20high-quality-care-kingsfund-feb13.pdf. Accessed 2018.

Year of Care Partnerships (2011) *Year of care programme report of findings from the pilot programme.* www.yearofcare.co.uk/sites/default/files/images/YOC_Report%20-%20 correct.pdf. Accessed 2018.

CHAPTER 7

Collaboration amongst professionals in primary care: examples from pharmacy

....

Elizabeth Mills

LEARNING OBJECTIVES

- Discuss the enablers and barriers to collaboration amongst pharmacists, other HCPs and patients in primary care.
- Describe a model for successful collaborative practice for the pharmacy profession.
- Provide examples of successful collaborative practice.
- Develop an action plan to increase collaboration with other members of the healthcare team.

Pharmacy in primary care in the UK has historically been limited to the lone pharmacist working in isolation in community pharmacy. Collaborations with other health professionals were few and far between. This was not through lack of desire to collaborate, or lack of understanding of the importance of collaboration for patient care, but as a result of a number of factors including the constraints of the pharmacy contract (e.g., lack of financial incentive to collaborate) and the legal requirements for a pharmacist to be present on the premises for the pharmacy to function. This inhibited the opportunity to meet and collaborate with other HCPs and engage with community groups. Bradley et al. (2008) have described the barriers to collaboration between pharmacists and GPs in the UK. These include the geographical separateness or isolation of community pharmacy from general practice and attitudinal barriers such as the 'shopkeeper' image of the community pharmacist. Community pharmacists were not generally viewed by GPs as a core part of the primary health-care team. In the UK this began to change with the large-scale reform of the NHS that began in 2000 (Department of Health, 2000a). As part of this reform the DoH in England recognised that pharmacy services needed to become 'integrated with other services' (Department of Health, 2000b). They laid out a vision where patients could expect to see pharmacists working more flexibly alongside other HCPs and outlined proposals to reform the community pharmacy contract to enable pharmacists to work more closely with other HCPs. In more recent years the increasingly complex needs of patients, ageing populations and shortages of healthcare workers such as GPs have led to a greater need for healthcare workers to take on new and expanded roles, and collaboration is key to tackling these new challenges. The following case study describes the Health Living Pharmacy Framework, which is an example of the reforms that have taken place in England to promote collaborative work between pharmacies and other primary healthcare services.

Case study: healthy living pharmacies

A Healthy Living Pharmacy Framework has been established which allows community pharmacies to deliver a range of public health services tailored to local needs. The framework is designed around three tiers of service provision. These are health promotion (Level 1), health prevention (Level 2, Providing services) and health protection (Level 3, providing treatment). The level at which services are provided depends on workforce development, the on-site premises and the relationships with other stakeholders such as GPs, social care and public health professionals (Firth, Todd and Bambra, 2015). Healthy living pharmacies are a hub for the community, catering for the public health needs of the local community.

You can find out more about the Healthy Living Pharmacy Framework from the following websites:

Pharmaceutical Services Negotiating Committee https://psnc.org.uk/services-commissioning/locally-commissioned-services/healthy-living-pharmacies/

Royal Society for Public Health www.rsph.org.uk/our-services/registration-healthy-living-pharmacies-level1.html

---

EXERCISE

- What barriers have you experienced when trying to work collaboratively with pharmacy in primary care?

There is increasing evidence from around the world that integrating pharmacists into a collaborative healthcare team improves patient outcomes. For example, Hwang, Gums and Gums (2017) report on the literature from the United States investigating physician–pharmacist collaboration on chronic diseases in the primary care setting, with a focus on hypertension and diabetes. In the majority of the studies pharmacists were managing medication therapy under the supervision of the physician. The pharmacists were undertaking activities such as assessing vital signs, reviewing laboratory tests, providing patient education, screening for drug interactions, identifying barriers to adherence and adjusting medication regimes. The author concluded that there was good-quality, patient-orientated evidence to recommend that physician–pharmacist collaboration should be considered as a way to manage patients with diabetes and hypertension. Law et al. (2013) describe how collaborative patient care is at 'tipping point' in the United States, citing an ageing population, chronic conditions and increasing costs of delivering complex care as the impetus for redesigning systems. In 2010, the International Pharmacy Federation (FIP) issued a policy statement on collaborative pharmacy practice stating that there is 'growing evidence of enhanced clinical benefit and good patient acceptability when pharmacists' practice is advanced collaborative practice' (International Pharmacy Federation, 2010). In the statement FIP recommend that collaborative pharmacy practice is promoted throughout the world and that each country takes steps to prepare their pharmacists and healthcare systems for collaborative pharmacy practice.

EXERCISE

- What are the benefits for your practice of collaborations involving pharmacy in primary care?
- How would the patients you serve benefit from collaboration with pharmacy in primary care?

The more recent focus of healthcare on person-centred care brings the patient into the heart of the collaboration. The House of Care model (Coulter, Robert and Dixon, 2013) assumes an active role for the patients and collaborative, personalised care planning. HCPs need to shift to a partnership model in which patients and HCPs work together using a collaborative process of shared decision making. HCPs need to learn to work together. Community pharmacists play an integral part in the House of Care model. In the UK, they represent a huge NHS resource. Of all, the NHS estate community pharmacists are the most numerous by number of cities and are located nearest to the population in a multitude of varied settings such as high streets, supermarkets, shopping centres and council estates; they are embedded in the community. Additionally they are open for extended hours, including evenings and weekends, and patients can access the pharmacist without the need for an appointment. Pharmacists are often in continuous and regular contact with the patient and have a holistic view of the patient's health and social needs. Community pharmacists should be essential team members in any patient-centred partnership model. The following case study describes an example of a pharmacy in London working collaboratively with the local community to provide community centred services.

Case study: the Wellfair Project

The Wellfair Project in West Euston is a partnership between Green Light pharmacy and a number of local voluntary organisations. Its aim is to improve the health and wellbeing of the local community alongside supporting local people to shape community services. As part of this partnership, Green Light operates a training programme for community volunteers which enables them to become community leaders on health issues. The pharmacy provides regular health education sessions in its purpose-built health educa-tion centre located in the basement of the pharmacy. The health education centre par-ticularly focusses on the needs of older people, ethnic minorities and people with LTCs.

The partnership has developed over a number of years since the pharmacy opened in 1999. The experience of the pharmacy in developing the collaboration is described in Table 7.1.

The strong links that Green Light has developed, with both the local community and other service providers including GPs, ensure they can be confident of providing the ser-vices the community needs (Department of Health, 2005).

EXERCISE

- Do you know how your local pharmacies are working with the community to deliver patient-centred care?
- Visit your local pharmacies to find out what services they offer and how they work with the local community.

The research into collaborative pharmacy practice in primary care mostly focusses on the development of collaborative working relationships between pharmacists and GPs. Developing collaborative working relationships with GPs is the first step to pharmacists becoming integral members of the primary care healthcare team. A review of the litera-ture on collaboration between physicians and pharmacists in primary care conducted in 2015 identified four specific models of collaboration (Bardet, Vo, Bedouch and Allenet, 2015). The Collaborative Working Relationship Model (McDonough and Doucette, 2001), developed in the United States, is the most cited model and describes the trust development between professionals in five stages: stage 0 – professional awareness; stage 1 – professional recognition; stage 2 – exploration and trial; stage 3 – professional relationship expansion; and stage 4 – commitment to the collaborative working rela-tionship. The drivers that influence movement along the continuum are defined as indi-vidual characteristics (such as age and professional background of each collaborating individual), context characteristics to do with the practice environment and exchange characteristics that relate to the personal exchanges amongst the collaborators (influ-enced by trust, role specification and partnership initiation). This is a theoretical model, although the drivers of collaboration are empirically tested.

The GP–Community Pharmacist Collaboration (GPCPC) conceptual model (Bradley, Ashcroft and Noyce, 2012) was developed in the UK based on research into collaboration between GPs and community pharmacists on local pharmaceutical services. It describes three stages to collaboration dynamics: isolation, communication and collaboration. The factors that influence the stage of collaboration are described as locality, service provision, trust, 'knowing' each other, communication, professional roles and professional respect. Figure 7.1 shows the GPCPC conceptual model.

The Pharmacist Attitudes towards Collaboration with GPs model (ATC-P) (Van et al., 2012) and GP Attitudes towards Collaboration with Pharmacists model

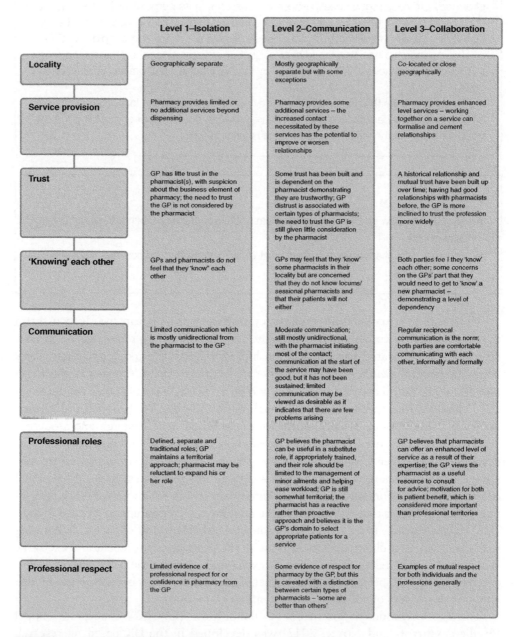

FIGURE 7.1 A conceptual model of GP – pharmacist collaboration

Source: Bradley, Ashcroft and Noyce (2012)

(ATC-GP) (Van et al., 2013), developed in Australia, are two empirical models that describe factors that influence pharmacist and GP (respectively) attitudes to collaborate with each other. Interactional and practitioner determinants of attitudes in these models include communication, trust, mutual respect, willingness to work together, clear roles, expectations, locality and previous experience contact with the other profession.

These four models, although developed through research in different parts of the world, have commonalities in the factors identified that influence collaboration. Table 7.1 shows a summary of these factors linked to a real-life example of collaboration from the UK.

TABLE 7.1 Factors influencing the extent of collaboration using the GPCPC model

Factor influencing the extent of collaboration (Bradley, Ashcroft and Noyce, 2012)	Examples from the literature	Example from the Wellfair project case study: the Wellfair Project
Locality	Close proximity amongst practitioner cites was found to enable collaboration, whilst distance was a barrier to collaboration (McDonough and Doucette, 2001; Law et al., 2013; Van et al., 2012; Van et al., 2013).	The headquarters for the project is in close proximity to the pharmacy, and the pharmacy, through the health education centre, is a delivery cite for services delivered through the project.
Service provision	In the GPCPC model, working together on a service was found to formalise and cement relationships.	Working with the community to provide community-centred services and actively support local community organisations with bid writing for funding grants has enabled a collaborative relationship to flourish.
Trust	Trust is a key factor in collaboration (McDonough and Doucette, 2001; Van et al., 2012; Law et al., 2013; Bardet, Vo, Bedouch and Allenet, 2015; Van et al., 2013). Gregory and Austin (2016) found that physicians and pharmacists based their trust on different cognitive models. For pharmacists, trust seemed to be based on status and position authority. For physicians, trust needed to be earned based on competency and performance.	Gaining the trust of the local community, through listening to their needs and being flexible in approach, was essential to develop a collaborative relationship in which the pharmacy is able to influence the services that are provided through the project.

continued . . .

TABLE 7.1 Continued

Factor influencing the extent of collaboration (Bradley, Ashcroft and Noyce, 2012)	Examples from the literature	Example from the Wellfair project case study: the Wellfair Project
'Knowing' each other	In the GPCPC model this was about the relationships with the individual CP and GP involved. This is reflected in other models as 'willingness to work together' (Van et al., 2012; Van et al., 2013), positive working relationships (Law et al., 2013) and relationship initiation (McDonough and Doucette, 2001).	Green Light described the need to take time to go out and meet the local community voluntary organisations and to find out how they work and what their needs are before any collaboration could begin. Essential to this is continuity of pharmacy staff involved in the collaboration, to be the 'face' of the pharmacy in the collaboration.
Communication	Regular two-way communication promotes collaboration (Van et al., 2012; Van et al., 2013; Law et al., 2013; Bardet, Vo, Bedouch and Allenet, 2015).	An essential part of developing the successful collaboration was being available for meetings and being accessible in between meetings. This is a challenge for community pharmacists delivering services within the pharmacy, when the pharmacist is legally required to be on the premises.
Professional roles	Shared motivation and working together for the benefit of the patient is more important than professional territories (McDonough and Doucette, 2001; Van et al., 2012; Van et al., 2013; Law et al., 2013; Bardet, Vo, Bedouch and Allenet, 2015)	Green Light and the local community voluntary organisations work together for the benefit of the community and adapt approaches according to need rather than professional role.
Professional respect	Mutual respect amongst collaborators and for the professions promotes successful collaboration.	Respecting the local community voluntary organisations and their ways of working has enabled successful collaboration to develop.

Source: Bradley, Ashcroft and Noyce (2012)

EXERCISE

Take some time to think about how you might collaborate with pharmacy in primary care to provide patient-centred care.

- Consider the stages of collaboration described in the GPCPC model. What stage of collaboration are you at with your local pharmacy services or community pharmacy?
- What are the factors that are currently influencing the stage of collaboration?
- What can you do to move towards Level 3 collaboration with pharmacy?
- What services could you collaborate with pharmacy to deliver to benefit patient care?
- Develop an action plan to move towards level 3 collaboration with pharmacy.

CONCLUSION

In this section I have presented a model of collaboration and discussed the factors that influence collaboration between community pharmacists and GPs. Examples of collaborations between pharmacies and the local community have been presented, with consideration of factors that have made these collaborations successful. Collaboration takes time and effort to develop, and the model presented is a useful guide to help focus these efforts.

REFERENCES

Bardet, J., Vo, T., Bedouch, P., Allenet, B. (2015). Physicians and community pharmacists collaborations in primary care: A review of specific models. *Research in Social and Administrative Pharmacy*, 11: 602–622.

Bradley, F., Ashcroft, D., Noyce, P. (2012). Integration and differentiation: A conceptual model of general practitioner and community pharmacist collaboration. *Research in Social and Administrative Pharmacy*, 8: 36–46.

Bradley, F., Elvey, R., Ashcroft, D. M., Hassal, K., Kendall, J., Sibbald, B., Noyce, P. (2008). The challenge of integrating the community pharmacist into the primary healthcare team: A case study of local pharmaceutical services (LPS) pilots and interprofessional collaboration. *Journal of Interprofessional Care*, 22(4): 387–398. DOI:10.1080/13561820802137005.

Coulter, A., Roberts, S., Dixon, A. (2013). *Delivering better services for people with long-term conditions: Building the House of Care*. London: Kings Fund Publications.

Department of Health (2000a). *The NHS plan: A plan for investment, a plan for reform*. London: The Stationary Office.

Department of Health (2000b). *Pharmacy in the Future: Implementing the NHS plan: A programme for pharmacy in the National Health Service*. London: The Stationary Office, p. 7.

Department of Health. (2005). *Choosing health through pharmacy: A programme for pharmaceutical public health 2005–2015*. London: The Stationary Office, pp. 27–28.

Firth, H., Todd, A., Bambra, C. (2015). Benefits and barriers to the public health pharmacy: A qualitative exploration of providers' and commissioners' perceptions of the Health Living Pharmacy framework. *Perspectives in Public Health*, 135(5): 251–256.

Gregory, P., Austin, Z. (2016). Trust in interprofessional collaboration: Perspectives of pharmacists and physicians. *Canadian Pharmaceutical Journal*, 149(4): 236–245.

Hwang, A., Gums, T., Gums, J. (2017). The benefits of physician-pharmacist collaboration. *Journal of Family Practice*, 66(12): E1–E8.

International Pharmaceutical Federation. (2010). FIP Statement of Policy on Collaborative Pharmacy Practice FIP, p. 2. Available from: www.fip.org/statements (Accessed 17.7.18).

Law, A., Gupta, E., Hata, M., Hess, K., Klotz, R., Le, Q., Swartzman, E., Bilvick Tai, B. (2013). Collaborative pharmacy practice: An update. *Integrated Pharmacy Research and Practice*, 2: 1–16.

McDonough, R.P., Doucette, W.R. (2001). Dynamics of pharmaceutical care: Developing collaborative working relationships between pharmacist and physicians. *Journal of the American Pharmacist Association*, 41: 682–692.

Van, C., Costa, D., Abbott, P., Mitchell, B., Krass, I. (2012). Community pharmacist attitudes towards collaboration with general practitioners: Development and validation of a measure and model. *BMC Health Services Research*, 12: 320.

Van, C., Costa, D., Mitchell, B., Abbott, P., Krass, I. (2013). Development and validation of a measure and a model of general practitioner attitudes toward collaboration with pharmacists. *Research in Social and Administrative Pharmacy*, 9: 688–699.

CHAPTER 8

Collaboration amongst professionals in primary care: examples from social work

....

Graeme Jeffs

LEARNING OBJECTIVES

- Summarise the legal and historical framework for social work practice in the UK.
- Identify some areas of collaboration between social work and primary care.
- Recognise examples of good collaborative practice in social work and broadly.
- Consider steps or actions on what might promote collaboration.

COLLABORATION: (NOUN) *'THE ACTION OF WORKING WITH SOMEONE TO PRODUCE SOMETHING'* (OXFORD LIVING DICTIONARIES HTTPS:// EN.OXFORDDICTIONARIES.COM/DEFINITION/COLLABORATION)

Social work is built on the ethos of collaboration between professionals and service users, between teams, across services and within communities. Collaboration in primary care is no different, but it brings some specific challenges. The author aims to provide some examples of ways in which social work and primary care can and do collaborate and how the challenges of collaborative work can be met.

AN ILLUSTRATION OF A PERSONAL EXPERIENCE

Firstly, a cautionary tale – I visited a department that at that time was developing a 'children's trust', bringing together separate teams into one seamless integrated organisation. The aim was to bring services and expertise together to share scarce resources, allowing families to get the help they need more quickly and with less duplication. During the visit, the managers waxed lyrical about the benefits of joint working. During a stop, the group had a tea break, and in the cupboard there were six jars of coffee all labelled with the different teams and separate shelves for each team's mugs and spoons: not to labour the point, but even if we work with the same people in the same building, that doesn't mean we are collaborating.

THE HISTORICAL, LEGAL AND STATUTORY BACKDROP

The relationship between social workers and primary care is predicated on the legal and statutory framework that social work operates within. This framework is particular to the UK because of the local legal context. The author summarises this context briefly to illustrate how this influences the types of collaboration that can and does exist amongst professionals working in a primary care context.

Social work and its origins

Social work as a profession deals with individuals, families, groups and communities, and its purpose is both to enhance social functioning and individuals' wellbeing.

Social work applies the findings of the social sciences – where it is taught as an academic discipline – and draws on thinking from the field of sociology, social policy, psychology, public health, community development law and economics to work with and between the networks that individuals live within and connect to.

The day-to-day work of a social worker is to conduct assessments and then deliver interventions or work with others to provide interventions to solve problems. These problems can exist on individual and community levels, and social workers move between these levels of influence to assist their clients. Social work, as with primary care in the NHS in the UK, is a universal service, not subject to eligibility criteria.

History

The discipline and practice of social work has its origins in the nineteenth-century volunteering and charitable works of Victorian England. The rise of social work is often seen as a response to the effects of the Industrial Revolution in the UK.

The development of social work as a profession is comprehensively covered by Horner (2003) and is not included in this text. However what is useful to note is that the gradual professionalisation of social work has contributed to an inherent tension between 'helping' those less advantaged and – as it seems with hindsight – patronising ideas of 'improving the poor'. These ideas are revisited in recent times in the debate in sociology around the rise of the 'underclass' (Murray, 1996).

Importantly, however, most social workers are employed by local authorities or voluntary organisations in the UK. They are rarely co-located with either the health or primary care workforce. They will therefore have different organisational priorities to attend to and possibly duplicative processes of assessment with primary care colleagues. Despite recent attempts, information systems for social care and healthcare do not easily talk to each other because of the different organisational boundaries, and families are often subject to repeated re-telling of their problems to multiple different professionals because of this fact. The 2018 cabinet reshuffle made changes to the civil service in the UK, rebranding the DoH to the Department of Health and Social Care, but this has yet to impact on the delivery of front-line services.

Regulation and education

In the UK, the Children and Social Work Act 2017 (Department for Education and Department of Health and Social Care, 2018) established Social Work England, a new non-departmental public body, whose focus is on public protection and ensuring quality within the social work profession, with oversight of the education of social workers.

There has been recent consultation to establish the legislative framework that Social Work England operates within. Its aims include the following:

- Setting profession-specific standards that clarify expectations about the knowledge, skills, values and behaviours required to become and remain registered as a social worker in England.
- Setting profession-specific standards for initial education and training to ensure that newly qualified social workers are prepared for the challenges of direct practice with service users.
- Ensuring that all social workers maintain their fitness to practice by setting out expectations for continuous fitness to practice and an operating a system to identify and support those social workers who are not meeting the standards.
- Having the power to set standards and approve and recognise post-qualification specialisms, helping to bring consistency to social work career pathways.

The education of social workers begins with a bachelor's degree (BA, BSc, BSSW, BSW, etc.) or diploma in social work or a bachelor of social services. Some countries offer postgraduate degrees in social work, such as a master's degree (MSW, MSSW, MSS, MSSA, MA, MSc, MRes or MPhil) or doctoral studies (PhD and DSW [Doctor of Social Work]). Increasingly, graduates of social work programmes pursue post-masters and postdoctoral study, including training in psychotherapy.

AREAS OF COLLABORATION

The most obvious way to describe areas of collaboration between social work and primary care is focussing on the main client groups social workers engage with and then draw out the relationship to primary care.

The primary client groups include the following:

- Children and families.
- People with mental health problems.
- People with learning disabilities.
- Older people.

Each client group has its own legal frameworks for social work and provides the wider context to social workers relationships both with their clients and other professionals.

Children and families

The social work role with children and families is primarily one of assessment, co-ordination and possible intervention, which can include a safeguarding element if needed. A social worker's role in assessing any child is described in legislation by The Children's Act 1989 (H.M. Government, 1989). Social workers receive referrals from GPs, schools, nurseries, and indeed local neighbours and family members. The key policy framework is provided by the 'Working Together' Guidance (HM Govt., 2018), which describes how services should work together to protect children.

Case study: working together to safeguard children

A social worker in a children and families safeguarding team is contacted by a local nursery. They are concerned about a four-year-old who has been with them for six months. The child's mother is sometimes late dropping the child off, she appears distracted, and the child is anxious. Recently he has appeared unkempt and hungry. Today he had a bruise on his arm. The nursery has tried to offer the mother support, but she appears uninterested. They know little of the child's background.

The social worker calls the registered GP and manages to speak to the receptionist, who offers to get the named GP to call back at lunchtime.

At this point the social worker is assessing the situation, and compiling information:

- Is the mother struggling to cope for some reason, and the bruise is a sign of over-physical chastisement?
- Could the family be in need of support and help, perhaps struggling with financial hardship? The bruise could be accidental, but nurseries rarely make a referral for no reason unless they have reason to be concerned.

Case Reflection

The reader might wish to consider how the relationship between the GP and the social worker might help or hinder an effective assessment of the child and his or her needs. What factors – personal, professional or organisational – do you think will affect the quality of service that will be provided from here on?

Recent policy directions are suggesting that mental health services' engagement with schools is a key area that would improve outcomes for children. Given that development, will the role of primary care and social work become more focussed on preschool partnership working? In a period of disinvestment from public services, might this be a sensible rationing of resources?

EXERCISE

- Think about any referrals you may have made to services. What were your expectations?
- What helped and what hindered you in understanding what would happen next?
- With hindsight, how could that process be improved for you as referrer, for the referred person and for the recipient of the referral?

People with mental health problems and older people

The social work role in mental health combines elements of assessment, treatment and risk management. The legislative framework in the UK is provided by the Mental Health Act 2007, which established the role of the 'approved social worker', the Care Act 2014 and also the Mental Capacity Act, 2005.

Social work in mental health has a rich tradition of partnership work, comprising the following:

- The idea of the multi-disciplinary team, managing mental health services in the community is firmly embedded.
- The growth of increasing access to psychological therapies (IAPT) has been an attempt in some ways to address the lack of resources to meet mental health needs that do not meet the severe end of the spectrum of problems.

There are clear generic elements of the social work role that are present in children and family work and in mental health: communication, planning, co-ordination and risk management. Effective IT systems sharing essential patient information are important, although the lack of single operating systems presents challenges for effective communication between mental health services and primary care. There is growing evidence that advancements in technology can help bring improvements in quality, efficiency, patient experience and, critically, in integrating health and social care (Kings Fund, 2018).

When considering what evidence we have about successful methods to develop joint working approaches in mental health, Felker et al. (2006) describe, through the lens of the depression treatment pathway, a three-phase process to improving collaboration:

1 Identify barriers to better depression treatment.
2 Identify target problems and solutions.
3 Institutionalize ongoing problem detection and solutions through new policies and procedures.

This focus on specific treatment pathways to promote collaboration might bring some benefits, move away from a broad aspiration towards collaboration and anchor the problem in the realities of service provision.

Older people

The social work role with older people and its link to primary care is of relevance. With the growth in LTCs, increasing life expectancy and complex comorbidities, the role of primary care in supporting health in elderly care has never been more high profile or more complex.

Rather than seeing older people as 'bed blockers' in hospital, and using social workers to have patients discharged quickly, the potential exists within integrated health and social care systems to use social work in a preventative role. As GPs develop better data on the stratification of their at-risk groups, the social work profession is well placed to support older people and their carers.

Family engagement is key to a social work approach and might mitigate the tendency of primary care to see individual episodes of illness outside the context of family, community, social isolation and deprivation. These could be complementary and not competing perspectives, but the challenge exists in how they should they be brought together. Co-location and commissioning of services at a population level might begin to address this, and recent interest in the ideas of the House of Care (NHS England 2019b) and support a focus on population health rather than individual illness.

EXAMPLES OF GOOD COLLABORATION

Honourable mention should go here to the long tradition of social work's inclusion in the child guidance movement and its development into Child and Adolescent Mental Health Services of today. The child guidance movement brought together educational psychology, clinical psychology, psychiatry, and social work and sought to integrate tertiary services for children, using a multi-disciplinary model of care. Often child development teams would be co-located with the child guidance team, bringing together the medical and psychological aspects of children's development and support for the benefit of the child. The predominant source of referrals for such teams would be from GPs.

In recent years, there has been a retreat from the integration agenda for children's services. Education is now focussed on standards of teaching in schools and less concerned with the 'Sure Start' model that underpinned the 'Every Child Matters' strategy of the 1990s and early 2000s.

EXERCISE

- What models of care might support collaboration? Consider the key elements of co-location, shared governance, a clear vision and focus on the needs of patients and families, and shared commissioning priorities which can be seen in the House of Care model.
- Which of these elements articulates the same sentiments but from a primary care perspective? This is the view from primary care looking from the inside out, whereas social care partnership work is viewing primary care from the outside in.

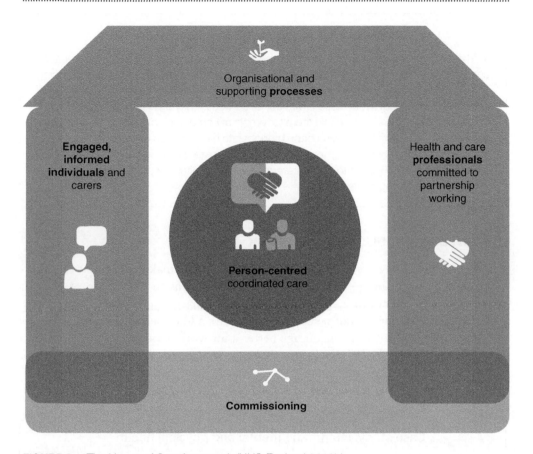

FIGURE 8.1 The House of Care framework (NHS England 2019b)

NEW MODELS OF CARE

The National Association of Primary Care (NAPC) identifies the 'primary care home' (NAPC, 2018) as another model of bringing together primary care and social care. Its model refers to the four ways in which primary care and social care coming together can benefit patients:

1 Information and advice, including signposting or referral to other services or support.
2 Care coordination, support for people with LTCs involving social as well as clinical needs – this might involve patients living in their own homes, residential care or nursing homes.
3 Advice from social workers on safeguarding, mental capacity and 'deprivation of liberty' issues in patient care.
4 Harnessing wider community resources and assets including the voluntary sector.

Case study: improving the co-ordination of care

In Thanet, four primary care homes have been established involving fourteen practices and a range of local health and social care bodies. An acute response team comprising a GP, nurses, healthcare assistants, physiotherapist, occupational therapist, voluntary care and care agency work closely with social services. They assess patients and put a package of care in place to enable them to remain at home or be discharged. Health and social care coordinators have also been brought into GP surgeries to provide non-clinical support to patients, and GP surgery hours have been extended to include weekends and bank holidays. This has led to better care outside of hospital, fewer hospital admissions and lower prescribing costs.

THE FUTURE MODEL OF SOCIAL WORK

The recent NHS Long-Term Plan (NHS England, 2019a) makes clear that the direction of travel for primary care will be broadly analogous to the House of Care or primary care home model. It specifically calls for primary care networks of local GP practices and community teams, supports them with additional funding and supports new organisational forms to encourage better joint work. Evidence of this approach is still emergent, but the following case study, drawn from the NHS Long-Term Plan, offers a flavour of the approach.

Case study: integrating mental and physical health

Covering all GP surgeries in Cambridgeshire and Peterborough, the Primary Care Mental Health Service ensures patients can access prompt advice and support for both their mental and physical health needs in a familiar community setting. The integrated nature of the service sees GPs, specialist mental health practitioners, recovery coaches, peer support, social care and third-sector staff working in partnership to provide overall care for the patient. The service focusses on people age seventeen to sixty-five with mental ill health. Promoting early assessment, treatment and onward referral in the community, the core specialist mental health service is provided by Cambridgeshire and Peterborough NHS Foundation Trust (CPFT).

A patient requiring routine, planned care or assessment will initially see his or her GP, who will seek advice from the Primary Care Mental Health Service or use an electronic referral system to arrange for the service to contact the patient. The service will arrange a face-to-face assessment or give the patient advice by phone. If they are in mental health crisis, they will be supported by the trust's First Response Service. The patient meets Primary Care Mental Health Service staff in his or her local GP surgery, meaning he or she is in a familiar environment and travel is reduced. Each GP practice in Cambridgeshire and Peterborough has clinical space for practitioners to run clinics on designated days during the week. Senior clinicians are also available to see people with complex presentations (NHS Long Term Plan 2019)

WHAT SUPPORTS COLLABORATION?

There are some tensions inherent in the practice of collaboration. A collaborative mindset would usually be a pre-requisite for a successful approach – this implies the ability to go above and beyond one's normal or usual role. For example, a social worker might normally see his or her role as solely a 'commissioner' of services and not a provider. In a field such as child protection, where the consequences of going beyond one's professional role can lead to damaging professional consequences and criticism, social workers may be forgiven for following a prescriptive or formulaic style of engagement with families.

EXERCISE

- What type of culture might a local authority safeguarding team need to create to foster a spirit of collaboration and yet ensure that social workers follow tried and trusted methods of working?
- What behaviour would one seek in a manager to support this approach?
- How might this culture differ from that of a busy GP's practice?
- Are they mutually exclusive?

We know however that some elements of job satisfaction come from a sense of clarity about one's role (Burton et al., 1980). The business of collaboration has at its core the ability to think outside one's own individual role and appreciate the contribution of others, perhaps adapting from one's own specific individual role (Phillipowsky, 2019b). How then do we conceptually reconcile the desire for certainty and job satisfaction and the need for exploration of collaboration?

WHAT SKILLS OR COMPETENCIES SHOULD BE ENCOURAGED?

Social services departments act as if they are in the domain of unsafe uncertainty, and their response, an increase in checklists, procedures, guidelines and regulations is to aim for the domain of safe certainty. The effect is that despair and depression set in amongst social workers such that many leave to take up other jobs. Checklists, guidelines and the like are useful but limited in the context of a belief of safe certainty.

True collaboration requires confidence in one's own skills, and happiness in a role comes from having some limits (knowing you've done your job well) but effectively managing anxiety about working across silos.

Suter et al. (2009), as part of a large Health Canada-funded study focussed on interprofessional education and collaborative practice, found two core competencies that support collaboration:

- Fostering the understanding and appreciation of professional roles and responsibilities.
- Communicating effectively.

For both these competencies there was evidence of a link to positive patient outcomes.

The author's personal experiences demonstrate social work has a role to play in the primary care environment. The exact role is still being determined as health and social care are brought together at a strategic level. What is also clear is that rigid pre-determinants of the relationships between social care and primary care can be broken down only by open and receptive collaboration. Collaboration in the eyes of the author, who uses examples from Mason (1993), who suggests that

> if we can become less certain we are more likely to become receptive to other possibilities, other meanings we might put to events. If we can become more open to, the possible influence of other perspectives, we open up space for other views to be stated and heard.

REFERENCES

Burton, G.E., Kundtz, R., Martin, G. and Pathak, D.S. (1980). The impact of role clarity on job satisfaction for hospital managers. *Hospital Topics*, 58(1): 12–18. DOI:10.1080/00185 868.1980.9954744.

Care Act (2014). Available at www.legislation.gov.uk/ukpga/2014/23/contents [accessed 01/08/2018].

Department for Education and Department of Health and Social Care (2018). *Social Work England Secondary Legislative Framework*. [online] Available at https://assets.publishing. service.gov.uk/government/uploads/system/uploads/attachment_data/file/713240/SWE_ Secondary_Legislative_Framework_Consultation_Response.pdf [accessed 20/05/18].

Felker, B.L., Chaney, E., Rubenstein, L.V., et al. (2006). Developing effective collaboration between primary care and mental health providers. *Primary Care Companion to the Journal of Clinical Psychiatry*, 8(1): 12–16.

H.M. Government (1989). *The Children Act*. [online] Available at www.legislation.gov.uk/ ukpga/1989/41/contents [accessed 13/04/18].

H.M. Government (2018). *Working Together to Safeguard Children*. [online] Available at www.gov.uk/government/publications/working-together-to-safeguard-children-2 [accessed 21/5/18].

Horner, N. (2003). The beginnings of social work: The comfort of strangers: Formalising and consolidating social work as a profession. In: N. Horner, ed., *What is social work?* 5th ed. London: Sage Publications.

Kings Fund (2018). *Digital Change in Health and Social Care*. [online] Available at www. kingsfund.org.uk/publications/digital-change-health-social-care [accessed 02/11/18].

Mason, B. (1993). Towards positions of safe uncertainty. *Human Systems: The Journal of Systemic Consultation & Management*, 4: 189–200, COLFTRC & KCC.

Mental Capacity Act (2005). Available at www.legislation.gov.uk/ukpga/2005/9/contents [accessed 01/08/2018].

Mental Health Act (2007). Available at www.legislation.gov.uk/ukpga/2007/12/contents [accessed 01/07/2018].

Murray, C. (1996). *Charles Murray and the Underclass: The Developing Debate.* [online] Available at www.civitas.org.uk/pdf/cw33.pdf [accessed 15/5/18].

National Association of Primary Care (2018). *Primary Care Home and Social Care Working Together.* [online] Available at https://napc.co.uk/primary-care-home/ [accessed 08/03/19].

NHS England (2019a). *The NHS Long Term Plan.* [online] Available at www.longtermplan. nhs.uk [accessed 15/01/19].

NHS England (2019b) House of care – a framework for long term condition care. [online] Available at https://www.england.nhs.uk/ourwork/clinical-policy/ltc/house-of-care/ [accessed 20/05/19]

Phillipowsky, D. (2019a). *Is This Integration or Assimilation.* Professional Social Work April, pp. 22–23. [online] Available at https://www.scie-socialcareonline.org.uk/is-this-integration-or-assimilation/r/a1C0f000006tJ37EAE [accessed 20/05/19].

Phillipowsky, D. (2019b). *Lead us in the Integrated World.* [online] Available at www.academia. edu/36638258/LEAD_US_IN_THE_INTEGRATED_WORLD [accessed 31/03/19].

Suter, E., Arndt, J., Arthur, N., Parboosingh, J., Taylor, E., and Deutschlander, S. (2009). Role understanding and effective communication as core competencies for collaborative practice. *Journal of Interprofessional Care*, 23(1): 41–51. DOI:10.1080/13561820802338579.

CHAPTER 9

General practice nursing in collaborative practice

Karen Storey

This chapter aims to describe how nurses in primary care settings (general practice) can benefit from collaborating with other nurses, GPs, practice teams, other professionals they interface with and patients receiving care. It looks at the benefits and barriers faced with adopting a collaborative approach in general practice and considers the advantages of this approach as primary care moves towards a scaled-up, integrated model of primary care networks.

INTRODUCTION

Major achievements since the 1990s have seen the UK General Practice Nurse (GPN) workforce evolve from playing a lesser and almost invisible role in healthcare to taking on a leading position in achieving the reforms required for the modernisation of the UK NHS. The evolution of the nursing profession has happened organically over the past decades and has moved away from being a task-orientated position to a key player within an integrated, multi-disciplinary primary care team (Redsell and Cheater 2008). GPNs have considerable autonomy in decision making; can take a history, make a diagnosis and decide on treatment options in conjunction with the patient; and prescribe medication. Many nurses are leading on developing new services and working with other members of the primary care team to develop different models of care and service delivery.

The expansion and progression of general practice nursing into advanced practice has raised the profile of general practice nursing and has given autonomy and increased decision making to nurses, putting their knowledge in some instances on a par with GPs (Horrocks et al. 2002). This is supported by a recent Cochrane Review (Laurant et al. 2018) of advanced nursing roles in primary care and suggests that care delivered by nurses, compared to care delivered by doctors, probably generates similar or better healthcare outcomes for a broad range of patient's conditions. Nurses in advanced roles have been seen to increase efficiency and streamline services whilst maintaining quality and improving patient satisfaction in general practice (Oliver 2017).

Investigations into the profession in recent years such as the DoH Work in Partnership Programme (2008) and Transforming Nursing for Community and Primary Care (HEE 2015a) have sought to examine the general practice nursing workforce. The introduction of competencies for GPNs by the RCGP in 2012 provided a framework to address the common core competencies and the wider range of skills, knowledge and behaviours nurses need to be a fully proficient GPN. The Primary Care Workforce Commission (HEE 2015b) highlighted the excellence as well as the challenges in general practice nursing and made recommendations which led to several policy changes to support the profession. Changes in nursing policy and education since the Shape of Caring Review (HEE 2015c) have helped transform general practice nursing with the introduction of a career framework for general practice nursing as well as opportunities for the Health Care Support Workforce to develop roles through apprentice routes and nursing associates into registered nursing. The General Practice Nursing Workforce Development Plan (HEE 2017) and the training hub networks developed by Health Education England in 2015 has seen a more coordinated approach to education and development for the profession with the rapid expansion of placements for undergraduate nursing students in general practice and the development of mentorship for GPNs.

In 2016 the Chief Nursing Officer for the NHS in England, Professor Jane Cummings (the professional lead for nursing), launched a five-year nursing framework for nursing midwifery and care staff (NHS England 2015) to support the delivery of the FYFV) (NHS England 2017a) In helping general practice to deliver this, NHS England launched the General Practice Forward View) (NHS England 2017b) with a dedicated action plan for general practice nursing. The 'General Practice Nursing Ten Point Plan') (NHS England 2017c) aims to recruit, retain and return nurses to the profession by 2020. It suggested how GPNs can play their part in contributing to address the challenges within the workforce and population healthcare by developing leadership skills and working more collaboratively. GPNs are vital to the forthcoming changes in the delivery of primary healthcare in England as policy focusses on general practices working together in federations and primary care networks and nurses working more closely in larger integrated teams. Opportunities for leadership, previously absent from general practice nursing, are emerging with the development of new roles in these organizations. The NHS England Long Term Plan (2019) advocates the development of primary care networks which focus on population health and prevention, provides opportunities for collaboration by encouraging GPNs, community nurses and public health and hospital nurses to work together for the benefit of patients, the public and communities. This direction of travel for general practice nursing is supported by the incoming chief nursing officer for NHS England Ruth May, who further supports the development of nurses in general practice.

The challenges in general practice

There are considerable challenges in primary care associated with ageing populations: increased prevalence of chronic and complex illness, multi-morbidity, increased demand on the system, diversity of the population and the outsourcing of so many hospital functions to the community (Roland 2014; Freund 2015). This complexity of issues means that often these cannot be solved by one single professional or profession (Samuelson et al. 2012).

Internationally it has been recognised that there is a critical shortage of GPs (Grover and Niecko-Najjum 2013). There are also considerable challenges internationally with recruiting and retaining nurses in general practice (McInnes et al. 2017). The nursing workforce issues are not widely recognised by the system or feature in the spotlight unlike the GP workforce challenges. The existing registered GPN workforce in England is ageing, with an estimation of one-third due to retire in the coming years (QNI 2015). With little or no succession planning, until most recently, this presents a nursing workforce challenge and potentially puts a strain on an already pressured system.

A large proportion of care for patients with long term conditions (LTCs) is delivered by nurses; a depleted nursing workforce could have a considerable impact on the delivery of care in general practice. This emerging vacuum for continuation of care for patients with LTCs and increasing work pressures on a disenfranchised nursing workforce means it is more important than ever before that general practice and primary care teams work collaboratively; the need for stronger interprofessional collaboration is essential to alleviate these pressures (Samuelson et al. 2012).

What do we mean by collaboration?

Collaboration in its simplest terms according to the dictionary definition is 'to work with others on a project'. Henneman et al. (1995) suggest that the act of collaboration is more complex and variable and can mean much more than just teamwork or cooperation, whether this is amongst professionals, with patients or clients. True collaboration involves having to understand the importance of equal involvement and shared ownership, mutual respect for each professional and their professions as well as individual expertise and opinions (Henneman et al. 1995).

Collaborative practice has been at the head of health service reform in recent years, and healthcare professionals have seen the value of collaborative practice in forms of teamwork and interdisciplinary and multi-agency work (Elsevier 2012). Interprofessional collaboration in healthcare has been described as 'an active and ongoing partnership often between people from diverse backgrounds with distinctive professional cultures who work together to solve problems or provide services' (Odegard 2006). Interprofessional collaboration not only increases patient satisfaction, patient safety and improved health outcomes but also increases team members' awareness of each other's roles and the knowledge and skills that each have, leading to improvement in decision making and patient care (Pullon et al. 2016).

Collaboration and teamwork amongst professionals has been shown to improve the quality of care, positive patient outcomes, improved efficiencies and satisfaction amongst professionals and has been shown to be one of the key elements in the delivery of cost-effective healthcare (Barrett 2007). However, other views link it to conflict, which implies that it is extremely complex and intricate (Jansen 2008). Teamwork and collaboration, whilst linked, the two have subtle differences in relation to leadership, power and autonomy (D'Amour et al. 2005).

When considering collaboration in general practice nursing, in an Australian study, McInnes et al. (2017) identified three themes common to the facilitation of and barriers to collaboration and teamwork between GPs and nurses working in general practice:

- Roles and responsibilities.
- Respect, trust and communication.
- Hierarchy, education and liability.

Facilitation and barriers to collaboration

The expansion of the general practice nursing role and sphere of responsibility has expanded in recent years but has often been perceived as supporting the needs of the GP role (Wilson 2002). Whilst GPs have been in favour of delegating workload to nurses, there has previously been concern by some doctors about the development of the 'independent practitioner status' (Koperski et al. 1997).

The historical power hierarchies between doctors and nurses exist; threats to the progression of nurses undertaking advanced practice roles include GPs perceiving these roles as a threat to their job status and concerns with the nurses' capabilities

(Wilson 2002). Barker et al. (2011) suggest that the differing views of what collaboration means, lack of interprofessional awareness, misconceptions about roles and scopes of practice and disregard for other professions provide barriers for collaboration. Collaboration is difficult to achieve in a hierarchy, which invests power in some professions and treats others as subservient (Fewster-Thuente 2008). The perception of physician dominance in decision making can be a significant barrier to collaboration as other professionals often do not have the opportunity to be involved in setting patient care objectives. Fewster-Thuente (2008) suggests that in true collaboration, hierarchy should not exist, and the knowledge of all professionals should be valued and taken into account.

Professionals working together should have an understanding of the professional cultures and stereotypes that exist as these historical beliefs, values, customs and behaviours distinguish one group of people from another and tend to be passed down from generation to generation (Hall 2005). Professional cultures and stereotypes allow people to establish themselves professionally and advocate for their chosen professions and, if not acknowledged, can often stifle opportunities for collaboration.

The unique, organic structure of general practice means, in most cases, that the GP who is the employer in the practice is considered the clinical leader and decision maker in the workplace (Burns 2009). Historically it has been suggested that GPNs have been seen as 'followers' rather than leaders and that the traditional clinical leaders in primary care have been GPs (Burns 2009). Effective clinical leadership involves complex interactions between leaders and the organisational environment that they wish to lead, and it is recognised that a good nurse–GP relationship is a significant enabler to leadership development and collaboration) (Mckenna et al. 2003). It has been suggested that a combination of organisational support, an enabling environment and an accepting culture appear essential to help nurses become aspiring leaders (Cook and Lethard 2004).

GPNs are often perceived as being professionally isolated from other nurses. Although they work daily with other nurses, they generally have closer working relationships with GPs (Crossman 2008). The nature of general practice work means that GPNs in England often work at a highly autonomous level, physical and professional isolation is often experienced, and many have no recognised support structure (Crossman 2008). Historically there has been a lack of teamwork, integration and skill mix and no effective workforce development in general practice nursing. In addition, the wide variation in access to training and development of GPNs has a direct impact on the levels of skills and expertise which affects the quality of care delivered to patients (Moger 2009).

The potential isolation and autonomous practice of nurses can result in confusion and misunderstanding of the legal implications for GPs in their role as an independent small business employer (McInnes et al. 2017). The degree of risk associated with this has previously caused confusion with indemnity and has been seen as a barrier to collaboration in practice (Condon et al. 2000).

EXERCISE

- Are these definitions of collaboration reflected in your current practice setting?
- What gets in the way of collaborative ways of working?
- What could you change to adopt a collaborative way of working with colleagues, teams and patients?
- How could you move from a dominant professional hierarchical mode to one of facilitator or shared leadership and decision making?
- Describe the advantages of having collaborative teamwork.
- Describe the disadvantages of not having collaborative teamwork.
- Consider the issues relating to facilitation and barriers for collaborative practice.

COLLABORATION IN NURSING

The Nursing and Midwifery Council (NMC 2018) highlights the importance of nurses working together with colleagues from similar and different disciplines. Collaboration is a broad concept including team functioning, respect, support for others, role clarification, leadership and conflict resolution (Mulvale et al. 2016). Whilst some professional groups have readily adopted collaboration, it seems the nursing profession has experienced difficulties in changing practice, and some have even resisted or rejected reform (Whitehead 2001). This may be due to the constant healthcare reforms and reconfigurations that have taken place in recent years. Collaborative practice forms the key to improving standards, nursing practice and future healthcare development. Implementing it into practice has been broadly absent in the profession as a whole, and as a result silo working has resulted from the lack of interprofessional coordination across the disciplines of nursing (Whitehead 2001).

The differing employment models in the UK for nurses have not helped foster collaboration and often form barriers amongst the nursing profession as a whole and increase silo working. Nurses working in hospitals and community trusts are employed by the wider NHS and are subject to the same employment, leadership and management structure. Nurses in general practice are usually employed directly by GPs who are independent contractors and have variable employment, leadership and management structure within each practice. Employment arrangements in general practice are widely variable, and this can mean that nurses are 'managed' by a GP or practice manager rather than by another nurse, although they remain 'unmanaged' in the traditional sense because there is no professional structure (Nutbrown 2003). Whilst efforts to address this are being developed and considered by general practice federations, CCGs and primary care networks through the introduction of general practice nursing leadership roles, this remains piecemeal across England. The opportunities that exist for integration in the new primary care networks will provide closer working for nurses and strengthen the need to invest in collaborative working.

LEADERSHIP IN COLLABORATIVE PRACTICE

It has been recognised that there is a lack of nursing leadership within general practice, which may account for the many issues that have been identified around collaboration (Cook 2005). General practices, in which nurses are able to develop leadership skills, are ones that have a culture in which staff offer each other mutual support, have a positive interest in performance, access to good communication networks and opportunities for professional growth (Buchanan 2003). The challenges are further compounded by the views from GPNs themselves who do not consider clinical leadership as a priority in their role and suggests the importance of developing such leadership skills is not always recognised by GPs or the nurses themselves (Hughes et al. 2006). However, the lack of leadership development has shortcomings, as GPNs' ability to influence situations within their practice is limited because they have no authoritative leadership role. Therefore, although GPNs might be assured that the workplace will provide opportunities for them to develop their skills (Norman 2005), there appears to be a need to raise awareness of the importance of clinical leadership development amongst GPNs themselves (Burns 2009). It has been identified that nurses empower their patients regularly, yet they do not empower themselves and cite significant barriers that contribute to this (Thyer 2003).

The lack of nursing leadership in general practice has an effect on both the quality of care for patients and on the organisational culture (Bondas 2006). Mckenna et al. (2003) in a study of community nursing, which has similar features as general practice nursing, identified that the traditional subservient culture of nursing is blamed for the perceived inability to nurture strong leaders and there is a reliance on leadership from GPs.

Case study: a triumvirate leadership programme

HEE, along with NHS Leadership Academy in the west Midlands, developed a primary care leadership programme in 2015, which includes a model of IPE known as a 'triumvirate'. The Triumvirate Leadership Programme is designed for the three key professionals: GPs, GPNs and practice managers from individual general practices attend the leadership programme together over a specific period of time. The programme allows protected time for the team to learn together and develop shared leadership knowledge and skills. The traditional hierarchical barriers that may have existed prior to participants entering the programme are challenged as the triumvirate teams discover professional, technical and other soft skills about each other that can enhance their working practices. Before the programme commenced, the organisations carried out a survey of the participants to see how they felt about aspects of their general practice. When this questioning was repeated at the conclusion of the programme, improvements were demonstrated in all parameters, including shared leadership (+16%), communication (+24%), organisational culture (+29%) and strategic vision (+23%). Four cohorts of the programme have taken place, and some practices have developed the model further by inviting other allied health professionals to join the traditional three, and clinical pharmacists, paramedics and other new roles have complemented the traditional team. This model is different from traditional leadership programmes, which aim to address individual's development needs and usually involve the individual attending a development programme away from the practice. The challenge then is for individuals using what was learnt in the programme and putting it into practice in the general practice environment on completion and on return to the practice. This approach requires time, effort and the individual's influence or position in the general practice team as well as persistence from the individual and often results in little or no change being made. The triumvirate leaders report that the impact of learning together in a classroom-based setting away from the practice with other triumvirate teams has brought about new learning but has also strengthened the professional relationships of the team. This gives them added confidence and influence to make changes happen on their return to the practice.

Despite the lack of leadership development and role opportunities nationally in general practice nursing, there are GPNs who have managed to take lead roles in practices and have advanced their skills and competencies to become independent prescribers, advanced nurse practitioners and partners in general practices, but generally the number of partners remains low (Cook 2005; Cernik 2007).

Case study: nurses as partners in general practice

Cuckoo Lane practice in Ealing London offers a model for nurse-led care; it aims are to provide high-quality personal healthcare and develop and maintain a happy multi-disciplinary practice which is responsive to patients' needs and expectations. The practice is run by two nurse directors and ensures that the team has a mutual participation model with patients so they're at the centre and can make decisions about their own care as much as is possible. The flat structure of leadership means it is not hierarchical, and there is a focus on teamwork. The practice has recently been awarded an outstanding CQC and was commended on the style of communication, leadership and collaboration between staff and patients. The unique model of communication is a twice-daily huddle for all members of staff – a briefing about what's going on that day facilitates collaboration. GP expertise is used in a different way so that they are employed in the practice for their medical expertise. Recognition of individual professionals' expertise and what all members of the practice can contribute encourages collaboration to flourish.

COLLABORATION AND CO-PRODUCTION WITH PATIENTS

According to a Kings Fund (2018) report, public satisfaction with general practice has declined to the lowest level since the National Centre for Social Research's British Social Attitudes survey began. Satisfaction amongst those sixty-five years or older was previously much higher than amongst other age groups; however, in 2017 satisfaction has fallen in all age groups, and one of the top reasons is long waiting times for GP appointments. The national GP patient survey provides more insight and reports so that patients are finding it harder to get through to their GP surgery on the phone, finding harder to see their GP of choice and rating their overall experience in general practice more negatively.

To deal with the complex healthcare and access demands of people, there are professionals in general practice who are looking at new ways of collaborating with patients moving away from the traditional consulting model to more innovative consulting models using technology and a concept of group consultations. GPNs in areas of England have embraced these opportunities to lead on and develop group consultations.

Case study: group consultation

GPNs in the North of England have been leading on a different way of consulting with patients. By changing the way clinicians consult, it shifts the balance of power, changes the clinical conversation, improve outcomes, creates time to care and improves both the patient and GPN experience.

Group consultations see ten to twelve people consulting with a GPN at the same time. All patients in the group have been invited and given their consent to participate in the programme and share their information with others.

Supported by a facilitator (often a healthcare assistant), the GPN joins the consultation after fifteen to twenty minutes once patients have looked at their results and thought of questions. The GPN consults one to one, with the other patients listening in and offering advice and support too. To understand the flow, go to: https://youtube/uZKVbKUvTfs.

Evaluation of GPN-led group consultation in the North-West found consulting with groups gave GPNs more time to explain and educate people. GPNs got to know their patients better, repeated less, had more fun and found clinics more fulfilling and energizing than one-to-one care. They also felt group consultations shifted the power dynamic, with the consultation being more focussed on the patients' than the clinicians' QOF review.

Patients benefit from better clinical outcomes – for instance, in seven clinical trials, patients' HBA1c fell more than usual care. They also gained confidence and improved their knowledge of their conditions. Satisfaction rates were high – at over 97%.

Case study: West Gorton medical practice, Manchester

As part of the North-West GPN Group Consultations Practice Development Programme, in 2017, Premiere Health and West Gorton introduced group consultations for adults with diabetes.

West Gorton calculated 100% efficiency gains in clinician time and saw eight to nine patients in the time it would have taken to see in a regulated four-minute-long one on one.

Across these two practices, thirty-one patients, followed up after three months, achieved an average 10% reduction in HbA1c (65 mol to 59 mmol/mol). In Premiere Health, six patients achieved an average reduction in blood pressure of systolic 12.5%

and diastolic 5%. In Premiere, the same six patients achieved an average weight reduction of 3.9%.

GPNs reported that group consultations shift the balance of power, are more person centred and support peer connection, with friendships forming from the first session.

Patients reported high satisfaction rates and learning more compared to one-to-one consultations even if their diabetes was well controlled. Some found group care less intimidating than one-to-one reviews. Staff found it time-consuming introducing group consultations. Staff learnt a lot from patients. Ninety-three percent of GPNs in this programme reported group consultations were fulfilling. No GPNs reported that they felt stressed or burnt out by group consultations, and 57% GPN reported that group consultations energised them compared to 19% describing one-to-ones as energising at baseline. Staff enjoyed consultations with less repetition. Group consultations accelerated Health Care Assistants and student nurse skills development where they were involved.

EXERCISE

- Take a few moments to reflect on consultations in your practice, what would it take to consider adopting group consultation in your practice?

CONCLUSION

The nursing role in general practice is an important and valuable contributor to the delivery of care to patients. GPNs in this role have now developed into a highly skilled, accomplished and essential asset in the general practice team. However, GPNs, as leaders and enablers in the system, require investment and support from GPs (as their employers) to promote their wider recognition as highly competent members of the interdisciplinary team.

Leadership that is shared and involves all members of the practice is integral to creating a motivated team. It is essential that nurses are supported to develop their leadership skills: without this step collaboration will not truly exist. Collaboration within general practice teams, and with professionals and others externally and across the wider healthcare system, requires a commitment from all to remove barriers, promote enablers and encourage mutual respect and professional confidence in each respective discipline.

REFERENCES

Barker, L., Egan-Lee, E., Martimianakis, M.A., Reeves, S. (2011) Relationship of power: Implications for professional education. *Journal of Interprofessional Care*, 25(2): 98–104.

Barrett, J., Curran, V., Glynn, L., Godwin, M. (2007) *CHSRF synthesis: Interprofessional collaboration and quality primary healthcare*, Ontario. Available at: www.cfhifcass.ca/

Migrated/PDF/ResearchReports/CommissionedResearch/SynthesisReport_E_rev4_FINAL. pdf. (accessed 25 June 2016).

Bondas, T. (2006) Paths to nursing leadership. *Journal of Nursing Management*, 14: 332–339.

Buchanan, D. (2003) *Leadership Organisations and Leadership Development*. London: NHS Leadership Centre London.

Burns, D. (2009) Clinical leadership for general practice nurses, part 1: Perceived needs. *Practice Nursing*, 20(10): 519–523.

Cernik, K. (2007) New opportunities for enterprising nurse. *Practice Nursing*, 18(11), 565–567.

Cook, R. (2005) Nurse partners: A quiet revolution. *Practice Nursing*, 16(9): 418.

Cook, M. J., Lethard, H. L. (2004) Learning for clinical leadership. *Journal of Nursing Management*, (12): 436–444.

Condon, J., Willis, E., Litt, J. (2000) The role of the practice nurse: An exploratory study. *Australian Family Physician*, 29(3): 272–277.

Crossman, S. (2008) Survey shows need for better access to training. *Practice Nursing*, 19(5): 249–251.

D'Amour, D., Ferrada-Videla, M., San Rodriguez, Martin L., Beaulieu, M.-D. (2005) The conceptual basis for interprofessional collaboration: Core concepts and theoretical frameworks. *Journal of Interprofessional Care*, 19(s1): 116–131.

Elsevier (2012) Inter professional collaborative practice in health care. *Getting prepared preparing to succeed, white paper* (accessed 8 November 2018).

Fewster-Thuente, L., Velsor-Friedrich, B. (2008) Interdisciplinary collaboration for healthcare professionals. *Nursing Administration Quarterly*, 32(1).

Freund, T., Everett, C., Griffiths, P., Naccarella, L., Hudon, C., Laurant, M. (2015) Skill mix, roles and remuneration in the primary care workforce: Who are the healthcare professionals in the primary care teams across the world? *International Journal of Nursing*, 52: 727–743.

Grover, A., Niecko-Najjum L.M. (2013) Primary care teams are we there yet? Implications for workforce planning. *Journal of the Association of American Medical Colleges*, 88(12): 1827–1829.

Hall, P. (2005) Interprofessional teamwork: Professional cultures as barriers. *Journal of Interprofessional Care*, 1: 188–196.

Health Education England (2015a) *Transforming nursing for community and primary care*. Available at: www.hee.nhs.uk/our-work/transforming-nursing-community-primary-care (accessed 8 July 2018).

Health Education England (2015b) *The future of primary care: Creating teams for tomorrow*. Available at: http://hee.nhs.uk/wp-content/blogs.dir/321/files/2015/07/The-future-of-primary-care.pdf (accessed 25 August 2018).

Health Education England (2015c) *Shape of caring review*. Available at: www.hee.nhs.uk/our-work/shape-caring-review (accessed 4 November 2018).

Health Education England (2017) *The general practice nursing workforce development plan*. Available at: www.hee.nhs.uk/.../The%20general%20practice%20nursing%20workforce%20 (accessed 4 September 2018).

Henneman, E.A., Lee, J.L., Cohen, J.I. (1995) Collaboration: A concept analysis. *Journal of Advanced Nursing*, 21(1): 103–109.

Horrocks, S., Anderson, E., Salisbury, C. (2002) A systematic review of whether nurse practitioners working in primary care can provide equivalent care to doctors. *British Medical Journal*, 324: 819–823.

Hughes, A., Elson, P., Govier, J. (2006) Developing practice nurses leadership skills. *Practice Nursing*, 17(8): 376–378.

Jansen, L. (2008) Collaborative and interdisciplinary health care teams; ready or not? *Journal of Professional Nursing*, 24(4).

Kingsfund. (2018) *Public satisfaction with the NHS and social care in 2017.* Available at: www.kingsfund.org.uk/publications/public-satisfaction-nhs-2017.

Koperski, M., Rogers, S., Drennan V. (1997) Editorial, nurse practitioners in general practice: inevitable progression? *British Journal of General Practice*: 696–698.

Laurant, M., van der Biezen, M., Wijers, N., Watananirun, K., Kontopantelis, E., van Vught, A. (2018) Nurses as substitutes for doctors in primary care. *The Cochrane Database of Systematic Reviews*, (7): CD001271. DOI:10.1002/14651858.CD001271.pub3.

McInnes, S., Peters, K., Bonney, A., Halcomb, E. (2017) *Understanding collaboration in general practice: A qualitative study.* Available at: www.ncbi.nlm.nih.gov/pubmed/?term=Fam+Pract.+2017+Sep+1%3B34(5)%3A621-626.+doi%3A+10.1093%2Ffampra%2Fcmx010 (accessed 11 June 2018).

McKenna, H., Keeney, S., Bradley, M. (2003) Nurse leadership within primary care: The perceptions of community nurses, GPs, policy makers and members of the public. *Journal of Nursing Management*, 12(1).

Moger, A. (2009) Improving standards in general practice nursing. *Practice Nursing*, 38(10): 40–42.

Mulvale, G., Embrett, M., Shaghayegh, D. (2016) 'Gearing up' to improve interprofessional collaboration in primary care: A systematic review and conceptual framework. *BMC Family Practice*, 17: 83.

NHS England (2015) *Five year forward view.* Available at: www.england.nhs.uk/five-year-forward-view/ (accessed 20 June 2017).

NHS England (2017a) *Leading change adding value: A framework for nursing, midwifery.* Available at: www.england.nhs.uk/wp-content/uploads/2016/05/nursing-framework.pdf (accessed 20 June 2018).

NHS England (2017b) *General Practice Forward View (GPFV).* Available at: www.england.nhs.uk/publication/general-practice-forward-view-gpfv/ (accessed 10 September 2018).

NHS England (2017c) *General practice: Developing confidence, capability and capacity: A ten-point action plan for general practice nursing.* Available at: www.england.nhs.uk/publication/general-practice-developing-confidence-capability-and-capacity/ (accessed 12 September 2018).

NHS England (2019) *The NHS Long Term Plan.* Available at: www.longtermplan.nhs.uk/wp-content/uploads/2019/01/nhs-long-term-plan.pdf (accessed at 10 March 2019)

NHS Working in Partnership Programme (2008) *General practice nursing toolkit.* Available at: www.rcn.org.uk/development/general_practice_nurse_toolkit/unit_one.

Norman, K. (2005) Leading the response to changes in nursing. *Practice Nursing*, 16(4): 189–190.

Nursing and Midwifery Council (2018) *The code: Professional standards of practice and behaviour for nurses and midwives and nursing associates.* Available at: www.nmc.org.uk/globalassets/sitedocuments/nmc-publications/nmc-code.pdf (accessed 24 May 2019).

Nutbrown, S. (2003) Practice nurses are unique. *Primary Health Care*, 13(6): 26–31.

Odegard, A. (2006) Exploring perceptions of interprofessional collaboration in child mental health care. *International Journal of Integrated Care*, 6(December), ISSN 1568–4156.

Oliver, E. (2017) *Advanced practitioners improve efficiency and patient satisfaction.* Available at: www.independentnurse.co.uk/professional-article/advanced-practitioners-improve-efficiency-and-patient-satisfaction/159765/18/10/2018.

Pullon, S., Morgan, S., MacDonald, L., Mckinlay E., Gray, B. (2016) Observation of interprofessional collaboration in primary care practice: A multiple case study, *Journal of Interprofessional Care*, 30(6): 787–794.

QNI (2015) *General practice nursing in the 21st century: A time of opportunity.* Available at: www.qni.org.uk/wp-content/uploads/2016/09/gpn_c21_report.pdf.

RCGP (2012) *General practice foundation: General practice nurse competencies.* Available at: www.rcgp.org.uk/membership/practice-teams-nurses-and-managers/~/media/Files/Membership/GPF/RCGP-GPF-Nurse-Competencies.ashx (accessed 22 January 2018).

Redsell, S.A., Cheater, F.M. (2008) Nurses' roles in primary care: Developments and future prospects. *Quality in Primary Care*, 16(2): 69–71.

Roland, M., Nolte, E. (2014) The future shape of primary care. *British Journal of General Practice*, 64(619): 63–64. DOI:10.3399/bjgp14X676960.

Samuelson, M., Tedesch, P., Aarendonk, D., de la Cuesta, C., Groenewegen, P. (2012) Improving interprofessional collaboration in primary care: Position paper of the European forum for primary care. *Quality in Primary Care*, 20(4): 303–312

Thyer, G.L. (2003) Dare to be different: Transformational leadership may hold the key to reducing the nursing shortage. *Journal of Nursing Management*, 11: 73–79.

Whitehead, D. (2001) Applying collaborative practice to health promotion. *Nursing Standard*, 15(20): 33–37.

Wilson, A. (2002) Barriers to developing the nurse practitioner role in primary care: The GP perspective. *Family Practice*, 19(6): 641–646.

CHAPTER 10

Collaboration and paramedicine

....

Chris Warwick and Stuart Rutland

LEARNING OBJECTIVES

- Evaluate the current and potential future roles for paramedics in primary healthcare.
- Appreciate the supervisory requirements for safe practice for patients.
- Understand the organisational requirements for true collaboration of the paramedical workforce.
- Understand international perspectives on paramedic activity.

INTRODUCTION

The role of paramedics in providing high-quality patient care in urgent and emergency situations through the UK 999 system is well established. Whilst the paramedic's professionalisation is relatively recent compared with other healthcare practitioners (College of Paramedics, 2017), particularly those with their roots in antiquity, modern behavioural changes in society – primarily in a 24-hour millennial information-rich generation – are shifting both the landscape of how patients access healthcare and their expectations of it. The paramedic workforce has rather naturalistically responded by capitalising on their capability and adaptability, seeking out opportunities beyond traditional work domains.

Challenges in maintaining a responsive primary care workforce, and recognition of the varied skill mix which can contribute to the best offer a healthcare system can provide to its citizens, have resulted in the opportunistic development of new and innovative roles for allied health professionals from a paramedical background. Increasingly specialist and advanced paramedics are to be found working in what traditionally might have been the domain of GPs and GPNs, providing front-line services to the unfiltered population when they seek healthcare input in primary care. In the UK, the Five year forward view (NHS England, 2014) and General Practice Forward View (NHS England, 2016) acknowledge the reality of the situation and the need to work collaboratively and develop existing HCPs to address the widening gaps in health and wellbeing, care and quality, and funding and efficiency evident in the NHS. The clinical and professional practice of paramedics is evolving predictably in response to constant and increasingly complex demands (College of Paramedics, 2017) as solutions to the challenges of increasing public tendency to call emergency services have led to the evolution of adaptable professionals with a skill set well suited to assessing, diagnosing and treating patients in the primary care setting and stratifying risk associated with often ambiguous presentations and with limited access to investigations.

CHANGING TIMES

The shift away from the perception of paramedics responding to patients who had experienced an accident or acute medical emergency, and concentrating on the need to respond rapidly, has emerged over the period since paramedics in the UK became governed by registration requirements in 2000, with the recognition that no more than 10% of their workload concerned high-acuity or critical presentations (South, 2012). As early as 2005, 'Taking Healthcare to the Patient' (Department of Health, 2005) described the UK DoH policy direction of ensuring that paramedics be equipped with a greater range of competencies to enable them to assess, treat, refer or discharge an increasing number of patients in the community. In response, ambulance trusts invested in a range of professional development programmes to upskill their workforce, with the ultimate goal of fewer patients being transferred to secondary care to address their health needs and access to diagnostic testing to make complex decisions in relation to their care – and the resultant reduction in costs, personnel and time that this approach engendered. The policy rhetoric remained explicit in the proceeding decade, and still both 999 demand and transferal to secondary care grew exponentially, suggesting that these new ways of working were either creating a dependence on an already over-stretched resource or that the system in which they work may not be best placed to deploy the paramedic as gatekeepers to secondary care.

In 2007 in the South East of England, the ambulance trust worked with the then Postgraduate Medical Deanery, the academic institution that oversees all training of GPs in the UK, to develop a 'paramedic practitioner' programme aimed at producing a pool of 'specialist' paramedics sufficient to ensure every patient accessing the emergency services, for whose needs may be better met at a location other than an emergency department, had appropriate access. A curriculum was developed in collaboration with local universities, the deanery and the local ambulance trust mirroring that of GP trainees in the UK in terms of process, leading to a postgraduate qualification for participants. The central tenet of the education was a two-month placement in primary care, where paramedics could develop, against a set of performance assessments, the essential communication and problem-solving skills to safely consult in a more patient-centred, risk-aware manner. The learning in this environment, which consisted of formal teaching in practice augmented with peripatetic and vicarious learning opportunities, was highly valued by the paramedic. Paramedics were encouraged to take responsibility when seeing patients in placement and discuss with GP colleagues through this development period, rapidly building both trust and recognition of the utility of the paramedic as a primary care practitioner. The role was benchmarked by a rigorous assessment of competence, namely, a large applied knowledge test and a circuit of fifteen 10-minute Objective Structured Clinical Examinations (OSCEs), all elements of which are written by high-performing specialists and advanced paramedics, using contemporary assessment and standard setting processes (modified Angoff) to underpin the assessment. The programme was positively evaluated and was popular with patients and professionals alike (Taverbie and Ruston, 2011), providing paramedics with, for the first time, access to work-placed education and development in a multi-disciplinary team that sought to capitalise on their experience as first contact healthcare professionals in the community. The adaptability and utility of the paramedic in primary care during this process was widely recognised, and as a result the profession began to transition away from exclusively working in ambulance services. This transition was further driven by ambulance trusts withdrawing such training and development opportunities and employees seeking out new opportunities elsewhere in the health service.

THE PARAMEDIC IN PRIMARY CARE

Less than ten years ago the only place that you would have seen a paramedic at work was if you had cause to call an emergency ambulance. The paramedic service provided was, and still is to a certain extent, predicated on the assumption that in accessing it, you are most likely seriously ill and as such need rapid intervention and/or escalation to definitive care. Whilst this is an important part of emergency service provision, in reality, with the absence of the community services that once supported patients to stay well in their own homes, 'calling an ambulance' has increasingly become the first resort for patients trying to access care in a quite-difficult-to-navigate urgent care system or where they have simply run out of alternatives.

This group of patients' needs are ill-defined prior to presentation, and as such they provide a dilemma to both the traditional paramedic service delivery model and the paramedics themselves, as to how best to manage them within a system that is safe for the paramedic, the patient and the employer. The modern paramedic has begun to adapt to manage these undifferentiated urgent care cases alongside the high-acuity critical care presentations, but a backdrop of increasing clinical complexity in an ever more challenging environment in terms of an apparent system-led reluctance to manage and stratify risk, rather than avoid it, continues to exert pressure on this workforce providing another source of pressure to an already heavily burdened workforce.

As a counter point to the millennial generation of care consumers serviced by both primary and acute care, the millennial generation paramedic has been emergent, demanding a career that is not bound to one employer or work environment. It is not uncommon for the standard ambulance-manning paramedic in the NHS today to work alone, with little tangible clinical supervision at point of care, and they will often be fearful of the repercussions of their practice in what is seen as a high-blame culture (van der Gaag *et al.*, 2018). Burnout and stress are high for this group of staff, and it is unsurprising that the paramedic profession has sought to develop and value relationships beyond those of the high-acuity specialist, forging new partnerships in environments where safe effective healthcare requires the generalist to manage uncertainty and risk within a system supportive of unanticipated outcomes and within a multi-disciplinary and empowered team. Given the high-pressure environment and intensity of work in the 999-emergency environment, modern paramedics can only be sustained to continue to deliver care in the NHS if they have future choices and career aspirations beyond the traditional 999 services. These choices are increasingly apparent with an efflux of paramedics particularly to primary care and weren't available to them as little as ten years ago, when their skills, knowledge and experience would have been lost completely to the wider health economy should they have decided to leave the workplace.

There is also a steep learning curve in terms of gaining experience in conditions I had previously not been exposed to very much in the ambulance service such as childhood illnesses or rashes. Having the ability to recognise those that need treating and the confidence to reassure parents when they don't is essential. I discharge patients autonomously much more often now whereas in the past I would refer the majority of patients for some kind of further assessment or care. A big part of this is being more comfortable managing risk and feeling supported in my practice.

Paramedic working in Primary Care, quoted with consent

EXERCISE

You manage a busy metropolitan GP surgery and, after the retirement of one of the senior partners, have identified that as a collective, you are struggling to meet the demands of all your patients. You have been unable to recruit a replacement GP and consider employing a paramedic for patients with on-the-day urgent care presentations and for home visits.

- Consider where will you advertise for this post and how will you make it attractive for the applicant.
- Where will you get guidance to ensure that the paramedic applicant will have met a standard that means he or she is competent to work in the environment?
- How much time will be put aside for the paramedic for clinical supervision?
- How will he or she add financial value to the practice?

PROFESSIONAL VULNERABILITY

The professional vulnerability engendered by the nature of 999 work and the reluctance of organisational systems to support the diverse nature of it is common in the paramedic workforce. Overcoming these vulnerabilities by valuing the adaptability, resilience, skills and experience of paramedics and wrapping them in an infrastructure that governs, supports and develops them and their practice has left them feeling less vulnerable and ultimately more capable, leading to the workplace as a secure learning environment being highly valued by the paramedic themselves. The careful support the transition requires to a specialist (yet definitely generalist) role in community paramedicine has been shown to involve various phases – a junctional 'decision making' phase then three 'active' phases, interwoven with categories: *engaging in a community of practice, adjusting to organisational and cultural change, developing critical thinking and mastering skills* (Long, 2017).

The transition and development of these abilities are easily identifiable by anyone who works in the environment as central to successful primary care delivery and more specifically the specialist in primary care, currently almost exclusively the GP. It is unsurprising then that the paramedic profession has begun to find a natural and synergistic home in general practice and wider primary care. At this early stage in their evolution, the key relationships for paramedics working in primary care are with doctors and nurses. As colleagues develop their own niches (outlined in the rest of this chapter), cross-profession working will need to develop to enable a seamless workforce, all of whom appreciate, value and respect each other's contributions and unique skill sets, to provide corporate, holistic care for patients. This becomes more pressing and important now that the paramedic profession in the UK has been granted, with appropriate development, prescribing rights across the full formulary (NHS England, 2018).

> …I'm constantly finding myself outside of my comfort zone. The team of GPs and practice nurses at my surgery have been incredibly supportive and welcoming, and the GPs take the time to progress my knowledge when I come across something unfamiliar. Although I have an unremitting sense of imposter syndrome, I also look back to when I first started, and realise how much knowledge and confidence I have acquired in that time. My professional autonomy is respected and encouraged, but equally, support is always there when I need it. It's extremely helpful to my practice to be able to follow patients up, and it has also taught me to make decisions for the best of the patient whilst balancing ambiguity and risk.
>
> Specialist Paramedic working in Primary Care, quoted with consent

DEPLOYMENT

Several models of paramedics in primary care exist already in the UK, and deployment appears to be variable and based on need: some paramedics will provide on-day responsive home visits only; others will provide surgery appointments, telephone consultations and specific clinics such as joint and soft tissue injection. A wide range of models are emerging which tend to be predicated on the needs of the local health economy and the adaptability of the paramedic. This highlights the urgent need for clearer definitions of what the types of 'specialist', 'advanced' and 'practitioner' paramedics' capabilities are, and the consensus appears to be emerging that these capabilities will reflect the adaptability of the professional and not be prescriptive but rather a standard that supports diverse and divergent practice.

Case study: breathing difficulty

A patient with a chronic respiratory condition calls you on Friday morning complaining of increased breathlessness; he calls probably three times a week and usually you are able to manage him over the phone without the need for a face to face consultation. You have a Specialist Paramedic who has just started at the surgery and you ask them to visit today because they have a relatively light clinic and few home visits. They visit and arrange a course of steroids and antibiotics and the patient calls you back on Monday to thank you for sending them around as they were very reassuring.

Case study: joint injections

You want to implement a joint and soft tissue injection service after a colleague who used to do this retired. A Specialist Paramedic has just started work with you and she is keen to develop within the role and is asking if she can be trained and run a clinic once a week.

EXERCISE

- Consider the potential issues raised by totally new groups of professionals joining the primary care workforce.
- How might this impact (positively and negatively) on patients' expectations and satisfaction?
- What efforts can we make to manage a change in expectations from patients about what types of professionals they might need to see?
- How can we make sure that we do not create a service that might be unserviceable into the future if we can no longer recruit paramedics?

ENABLERS

Tangible clinical supervision and multi-disciplinary teamwork appear to be the key enablers to facilitate practice in this environment and at the level described in the case studies. In a well-led GP surgery, this feels very much like the GPs as consultants of primary care with a team of capable generalists around them supporting the delivery of that care. Mature capability frameworks that link to validation, cyclical appraisal and revalidation amongst the peer group are essential here. The two case studies reflect positive outcomes; however, consider each if the outcome had been negative. The patient's narrative may have been wholly different; however, the outcome may have been the same regardless of the clinician who saw those patients. Enabling the paramedic to practice without constant affirmation and validation from medical colleagues liberates them but does require some careful consideration as to the implications of practice at this level.

EXERCISE

- How can clinical supervision be provided safely and effectively for paramedics in primary care?
- How will you ensure that the paramedic does not increase your workload by relying on you to make all of the decisions in relation to patient care?
- How will you ensure that quality clinical care has been and continues to be delivered when patient outcomes are unanticipated?
- What about educational supervision? Does professional identity affect the ability to provide meaningful career development support?

TRAINING AND EDUCATION NEEDS FOR PARAMEDICS TO WORK SAFELY IN PRIMARY CARE

Paramedic education and training have developed rapidly in recent years, moving from a brief introduction to emergency management to a system in which an undergraduate degree is now the minimum entry point (Allied Health Solutions, 2013). Those paramedics with extensive experience, but no degree, bring wisdom and insight but require appropriate career development options to contribute to the expanding roles required in a more collaborative primary care environment. In the UK, local systems have developed to support and certificate this, and efforts to define national standards are ongoing. Transferability of competences, and capabilities, is increasingly important with a mobile workforce of professionals, much less likely than previous generations to live out their entire working lives with one or two employers. Higher education establishments (HEIs) are rising to this challenge, developing Level 7 (master's) programmes catering for those practitioners who wish to expand their skills to take on the roles we have discussed. Professional bodies such as The College of Paramedics are also embracing these new ways of working by providing threshold entry exams using established contemporary assessment methodology to registers of extended clinical practice.

COLLABORATION BEYOND JOINING THE TEAM

Examples of improved collaboration between paramedic services and primary care demonstrate that benefits are available beyond the traditional practice-based model of care. By creating a workforce with extended scope of practice (ESP) in Canada (Stirling et al., 2007), case studies have shown increased interactions between ambulance services and rural communities with an overall benefit to healthcare through increasing community response capacity, linking communities more closely to ambulance services and increasing health promotion and illness prevention work at the community level. As with all professions, leadership, management, problem solving and communication skills are important for paramedics to successfully undertake expanded scope roles. The report concluded that ESP in rural locations can improve healthcare beyond direct clinical skill by active community engagement that expands the capacity of other community members and strengthens links between services and communities. As health services look to gain maximum efficiency from the health workforce, understanding the intensification of effort that can be gained from practitioner and community coalitions provides important future directions (Stirling et al., 2007). A Canadian systematic review confirmed that ESP paramedics can safely contribute to community healthcare provision (Bingham et al., 2012). Similar care models, focussing on reduction in transport to emergency departments, have been shown around the Western world to be safe, effective and economically sound (Hoyle et al., 2012). The New Zealand perspective highlighted the potential for mindful prioritisation of dispatch to maximise effectiveness of their approach.

Case study: virtual wards

Rural areas in the UK are taking things further, with NHS Lanarkshire developing their Age Specific Service Emergency Team (ASSET) for frail and elderly patients. A 'virtual ward' backs up the service, provided by paramedic practitioners, enabling specialist care in the patients' own homes (Scottish Ambulance Service, 2015). For care to move closer to home, such services need to proliferate elsewhere through proper commissioning, and the intention is for an autonomous service collaborating with all the other elements of the NHS in Scotland.

CONCLUSION

In the UK the move towards paramedicine contributing significantly to the primary care workforce has been more borne out of challenges to recruit more traditional roles than by joined-up strategic thinking by policymakers. Like the best organic situations, it has contributed to revitalising the career options for a whole new professional group that may previously have been lost to the NHS and shows no signs of abating. Primary care systems which fail to appreciate the vital contribution paramedics can bring do so at their peril.

One consequence of the burgeoning community of paramedic practitioners has been potentially to destabilise the traditional emergency response services, with preferable working hours and conditions to be exploited by paramedics seduced by struggling practices keen to recruit any appropriate professional to maintain their patient care commitment. New rotational models of working, with paramedics spending equal periods moving through placements in the acute ambulance trust, general practice and other community settings appear to offer opportunities to maintain a generalist and comprehensive skill set whilst supporting three key sectors in the provision of urgent and emergency care (Health Education England, 2018). Whether such rotational posts will prove attractive to professionals remains untested. The risk without such measures, as with all shifts of individuals in any healthcare system with significant vacancies, is that attempts to modernise and support one area of the offer for patients is made at the expense of another. Collaboration at the system level is therefore essential to ensure the provision as a whole meets patients' needs whilst responding to the paramedics ambitions and aspirations.

REFERENCES

Allied Health Solutions (2013). Paramedic Evidence Based Education Project (PEEP) end of study report (Online). Available from: www.collegeofparamedics.co.uk/downloads/PEEP-Report.pdf (Accessed 28 May 2018).

Bingham, B.L., Kennedy, S.M., Drennan, I. and Morrison, L.J. (2012). Expanding paramedic scope of practice in the community: A systematic review of the literature. *Prehospital Emergency Care*, (3): 361–372.

College of Paramedics (2017). *Paramedic Post-Graduate Curriculum Guidance*. College of Paramedics, Bridgwater.

Department of Health (2005). *Taking Healthcare to the Patient: Transforming NHS Ambulance Services*. Department of Health, London.

Health Education England (2018). Paramedics (Online). Available from: https://hee.nhs.uk/our-work/paramedics (Accessed 28 May 2018).

Hoyle, S., Swain, A.H., Fake, P. and Larsen, P.D. (2012). Introduction of an extended care paramedic model in New Zealand. *Emergency Medicine Australasia*, 24(6): 652–656.

Long, D. (2017). Out of the silo: A qualitative study of paramedic transition to a specialist role in community paramedicine (Online). Available from: https://eprints.qut.edu.au/114997/ (Accessed 28 May 2018).

NHS England (2014). Five year forward view (Online). Available from: www.england.nhs.uk/wp-content/uploads/2014/10/5yfv-web.pdf (Accessed 30 April 2018).

NHS England (2016). General practice forward view (Online). Available from: www.england.nhs.uk/publication/general-practice-forward-view-gptv/ (Accessed 30 April 2018).

NHS England (2018). Paramedic prescribing (Online). Available from: www.england.nhs.uk/ahp/med-project/paramedics/ (Accessed 28 May 2018).

Scottish Ambulance Service (2015). Towards 2020: Taking care to the patient (Online). Available from: www.scottishambulance.com/UserFiles/file/TheService/Publications/Strategic%20Plan_Online%20pdf.pdf (Accessed 28 May 2018).

South, A. (2012). Right care, right place, right time? *Journal of Paramedic Practice*, 4(2): 67.

Stirling, C.M., O'Meara, P., Pedler, D., Tourle, V. and Walker, J. (2007). Engaging rural communities in health care through a paramedic expanded scope of practice. *Rural and Remote Health*, 7(4): 1–9.

Taverbie, A. and Ruston, A. (2011). An evaluation of a training placement in general practice for paramedic practitioner students: Improving patient-centred care through greater inter-professional understanding and supporting the development of autonomous practitioners. *Quality in Primary Care*, 19(3): 167–173.

van der Gaag, A. and Jago, and Austin, Z., Zasada, M., Banks, S., Gallagher, A. and Lucas, G (2018). Why do paramedics have a high rate of self-referral? *Journal of Paramedic Practice*, 10(5): 205–210.

CHAPTER 11

Concluding remarks on collaborative primary care

Sanjiv Ahluwalia, Karen Storey and John Spicer

In this chapter we will draw the central themes that the authors and contributors have highlighted as salient to the provision of collaborative care in primary health. It remains to review what are the most important and how they may play out in the future: this is the content of the final chapter. Drawing together these themes and how they are interpreted by the professional groups identified, the following seem contingent.

PROFESSIONAL EDUCATION

Fundamentally, the reason to engage with a discussion on best collaborative care is only important if it improves the lot of both patients and health and social care workers. To that end, and especially in the community, we accord the role of education as central. Both at the qualifying level (otherwise known as *pre-certification* or *undergraduate* or other synonyms) and at the continuing education (or professional development) phase, it is clear that those who learn together practice better together. Further, this is likely to hold for those staff who do not have a formal certification or regulated status. The value of such IPE is multiple – improving the care of patients, it also permits the evolution and legitimation of professional and clinical identity and acceptance of as such by members of a team. IPE provides the right environment to explore the boundaries, governance and limitations of professionals' roles to develop an appreciation and understanding that is required in a system-based care setting. That there is still work to do is explored by Griffin and O'Keeffe in some detail in their chapter and remains an issue around the world (Wong, 2018).

THEORY AND EVIDENCE IN PRIMARY CARE

One of the traditions of the apprenticeship model of learning is that it can be overly focussed on occupational preparation (Billet, 2016) and less so on the theories that underlay practice. In community practice the need for a commonality of theory and practice has never been greater (Allan et al., 2018). That theory could be the evidence base in, for example, clinical outcomes by treatment but should also exemplify conceptual issues in community care. Such an approach, it could be argued, will only enhance collaborative care. The evidence base in generalist care is more limited than in specialist care for many reasons but particularly because of the complexity of the community-situated patient under the care of a multi-professional team. Theoretical approaches to the functioning of community teams can be founded on empirical evidence too, and several studies have approached this, not always with a clear outcome (Körner, 2016), but studies can suggest some of the pre-requisites for good multi-professional collaboration (Sorensen et al., 2018; Van Loenen et al., 2016).

PROFESSIONAL IDENTITY

The functioning of the primary care team as a dynamic organisation is crucial to the good delivery of its product. All our authors have described this in various ways. That team members should share similar values may appear unreservedly optimistic, but they might be held to exist in a certain *ecology* of factors and pressures (Pattison and Pill, 2004). This means a mutual respect amongst team members is easier to achieve, and it is clear that such a respect will engender its better functioning. Each profession can claim a certain professional identity, although it is arguably more historically developed in some (e.g., doctors) than others (e.g., paramedics). Such an imbalance may reduce the mutual respect important in establishing collaborative practice. So those disciplines whose professional identity is in some sense emergent may have everything to gain from working in good multi-disciplinary teams. That said, professional groups do tend to see collaborative practice in similar ways, and perhaps that represents a commonality of values. In fact, Machin et al. (2018) describe a need for a shared moral language to underlie the collaborative enterprise of team-based care, a consideration with which we would not disagree and share their educational approaches to foster such a language.

TEAMS

Teamwork is where different people of a team or group work together under any circumstances, offering constructive feedback and using their own skills, no matter what kind of personal relationships they may otherwise be sharing. Most of the time teams have a strong leader who has the authority to solve disputes and coordinates actions. The leader plays an important role, and he or she has a strong responsibility to help make a team successful. The result of teamwork or collaboration is usually the same. When there is collaboration in a group, they are working together to reach a goal. Each member of that group shares the same vision. This is also what happens in teamwork; the members of this group also work towards reaching a certain goal. Traditionally teams in general practice are small and close-knit; however, with the introduction of larger integrated primary care, working teams can become bigger and have less-defined structures (Pettigrew et al., 2019)

Effective teamwork relies on effective communication amongst the team members, and the lack of communication in the workplace affects teamwork and patient outcomes (Hallin et al., 2011). Communication does not always work effectively, and lack of communication affects collaborative practice (Hallin et al., 2011). Mickan and Rodger (2005) offer the following as being essential to successful teamwork:

- Common purpose.
- Measurable goals.
- Effective leadership.
- Effective communication.
- Good cohesion.
- Mutual respect.

Woven throughout this book are illustrations of team-based work in which these elements are displayed if not explicitly described. Given the tight-knit nature of small primary care teams, these characteristics are not only essential to engender but also must be maintained to deliver high-quality services.

SPACES IN WHICH TO COLLABORATE

What is sometimes known as *estate* is humdrum but cannot be ignored. Although the work of primary or community care teams is often conducted at the home of the patient, mostly it is done in a dispersed network of buildings around a given area. It is not conveniently located within the four walls of a hospital. This can make it difficult for team members to come together to exercise their function. In reality it is even more complicated than that: buildings are simply the space within which clinicians and business managers work. The ways the people and the buildings are clustered into organisations that function, and control the money flows that make it happen or indeed relate to the communities they collectively serve is of immense importance. These structural issues cannot but affect the work of the team (Gunn, 2015). With some exceptions this arena has not received the notice it should have done, and certainly the workplaces that primary and community teams need to work collaboratively have not either (Bailey et al., 2018). We argue that collaborative care should have access to modern facilities suitable for clinical practice (generally the only quality in regard by funding agencies in the UK), interprofessional development, teaching and learning, and community engagement.

TECHNOLOGY IN PRIMARY CARE

Issues of space and context are relevant to the quality of care delivered in primary care. They are also relevant to the provision of education and formation of professional identity. It is perhaps not controversial to acknowledge (at the time of writing this chapter) that certain professional groups hold sway on the management and dispersal of resources, access to educational opportunities and collective bargaining to influence healthcare policy. This is of particular relevance to 'newer' members of primary care teams at a time when such teams are becoming more diverse and more comprehensive in their skills (Woodson et al., 2018). All our contributors acknowledge these differences and how technology might offer solutions. From democratising knowledge, connecting people and teams in new virtual spaces, and offering solutions to working with patients, technology offers the greatest potential to re-shape the balance of power and identity amongst the professions. Working in collaboration to modernise our healthcare service offers the greatest chance of success in improving patient outcomes and resulting in meaningful careers. It is also worth noting that the delivery of good care, enhanced by collaborating teams, also requires the explicit engagement of patients (Castle-Clarke and Imison, 2016).

ASSET-BASED APPROACHES TO COMMUNITY DEVELOPMENT

A number of the authors in this book allude to the difference between 'the community' and hospitals as spaces for providing care. Whilst we have briefly explored the nature of space and context in the previous paragraph, one item merits further mention. Many of our authors also describe the value and importance of asset-based approaches to community development, especially when health and social care engage with third and voluntary sector organisations in planning and delivering care. *GPs in the Deep End* (Watt, 2012), social prescribing and other navigation strategies, connections with housing and employment services through to influencing local policy on green spaces and other environmental issues – these are all examples of the power and importance of successful collaboration arising from primary care. Group consultations are a method of asset-based community development as it utilises the assets in the patient community as an empowered self-organising collective.

For the reader, we also draw the distinction between asset-based community development (Chana & Ahluwalia, 2014) and other forms of managerial and policy intervention. Whilst standard approaches to 'problems' (whether these be in primary or secondary care) is to identify the problem, search out solutions and measure improvements till the problem has been resolved, asset-based community development takes a different route. It starts with identifying the areas of strength and opportunities for harnessing energy that exist in a community. Both approaches start in very different ways of thinking: traditional approaches work well for clearly defined, measurable and time-context limited issues; asset-based approaches are better suited to understanding and engaging with those messy situations often seen in communities. Many of our authors recognise this distinction and draw on the value of empowerment through collaboration to improve care for their patients in primary care, recognising that they are key elements within the complex and messy world that sits outside hospitals.

LEADERSHIP FOR COLLABORATION

Historically leadership in primary care has been a hierarchical structure where the GP who was the owner of the practice was the nominated leader who made both clinical and business decisions. A hierarchical structure does not work in collaboration, and traditional forms of leadership are a barrier to its success. Our authors clearly describe a shift in primary care and general practice from traditional hierarchical leadership to newer models of shared or collective leadership. Shared or collective leadership in collaboration is an endeavour that requires all members of the group to participate.

In times of danger it can be highly advantageous to have one leader and one voice to lead on decision making. However, in the day-to-day workings of primary care, this is not needed, and having collective leadership from many members of the team brings a variety of perspectives, experiences and skills. Multi-professional leadership within a group or team makes for better decision making (West et al., 2014). The lack of nursing and other allied health professional leadership development in primary care in previous years has now been acknowledged, and efforts are underway to tap into the wealth of high-quality leadership dormant within general practice teams and groups.

The characteristics of leadership to support collaborative practice in primary care include influencing skills, self-awareness of different styles, being goal oriented, promoting collective responsibility for achieving improved clinical outcomes, agnostic to the position or employment status of individuals involved in providing care, working as part of informal as well as formal arrangements and accepting collective responsibility for the success of the organisation, not just for professionals own jobs or areas.

West goes on to say that in cultures where there is collective leadership, all staff members will intervene to solve problems to improve quality of care and create supportive environments that in turn result in positive outcomes for patients. As discussed by the collective authors, collaboration relies on relationships and a lot of give and take amongst the participants, so collaboration and teamwork, no matter how similar they may seem, are different and work differently but help produce the same result, reaching a goal together that proves beneficial for organisations and is conducive to its growth. Collaboration is often mistaken as teamwork as it often requires many people to work on a project together. Although there is a certain element of teamwork here, it is different, and instead of calling it a team, it would rather be wise to refer to it as collective. Instead of having a group of people performing their individual tasks to reach a goal, in collaboration, there is a group of people creating a collective mind to reach a goal or solve a problem.

JOURNEYS AND JOBS

Recruitment and retention of the workforce into primary care is a challenge facing all healthcare systems across the globe (Roland, 2015). Mutual respect for each other spurs a sense of both belonging as well as professional development. But most importantly, collaborating offers the opportunity to reframe careers in primary care not as roles fixed for decades but as journeys that are to be experienced and where individuals evolve over a period of time.

The competitive spirit (seen in procurement and commissioning as policy levers) pits professionals against each other and ultimately away from the needs of our patients and communities – it renders our relationships and interactions as adversarial, emotionally draining and limiting. Repeated iterations of the purchaser–provider split highlight that primary care loses to other sectors but particularly secondary care – the workforce is demoralised and impoverished. Collaboration is the perfect antidote – it replaces the negativity associated with adversity with a sense of purpose and energy that has the potential to make primary care an attractive place to work. Primary care has the potential to become a life's journey, not just another job. The rewards are all the more powerful for improving patient outcomes given the evidence that a happier workforce results in better patient care (West and Dawson, 2012).

RESOURCES AND CARE

Primary care has been at the forefront of making do with remarkably little. Current spending on primary care is less than 10% but provides 90% of contacts in the NHS. A key to achieving this is that funding for primary care is capitated – it is based on a fixed budget, and practices must manage to provide high-quality care within resources. There is no 'bailout' for over-performance in primary care. A key to the success of primary care in managing resources has been a strong need to collaborate (within teams, with patients and with local communities) as well as innovation. It is perhaps not surprising that the move towards larger organisations in primary care and contract reform has been slow – the ability of primary care to absorb clinical and financial risk, continuously evolve and remain relevant to the populations it serves are recognised as fundamental to the stability of the NHS.

Indeed, recent UK healthcare policies are keen to build upon the model of general practice with its list-based capitated funding model to develop integrated care systems. For integrated care systems to be successful, they will require collaboration at their heart, innovation driven to improve quality and reduce cost, and a shift towards prevention that is unprecedented in the history of the NHS.

It remains to be seen how the tensions between collaboration and procurement will influence the health and care system over the coming decade. It also remains to be seen if integrated care systems can develop the maturity required to successfully embed collaboration at the heart of their functioning. What we think is clear is that without promoting collaboration over marketised means and investment in prevention and public and population health, it is likely that integrated care systems will struggle to achieve the 'holy trinity' of improved patient experience, better quality care and reduced costs.

INVOLVING PATIENTS AND COMMUNITIES

We end this chapter (and the book) with perhaps the most important ingredient woven throughout – collaboration with patients and their communities. Primary care occupies the same physical and ecological space as patients – a unique success of primary care is that it is as close as possible to where people live; the challenge for the next generation must be to determine how we can improve the resilience and range of services for patients without compromising the spaces that exist for them to access their care and needs. How we move to larger practices and networks alongside the wish of patients to be able to access spaces close to their lives is a challenge that will unfurl over the coming time.

What is certain, though, is that without engaging patients in their care as well as how services are delivered, we will never achieve the combined desire for high-quality and improved outcomes. Collaboration with our patients (and their communities) is therefore paramount. Many of the authors in this book describe the centrality of engagement and collaboration with patients and communities, and primary care has a well-developed set of arrangements for doing so. But there is so much more to do – how can primary care reach out to those who are disadvantaged and without voice; how does primary care seek to dent the ingrained inequalities described by Tudor-Hart (Appelby and Deeming 2001); and how can primary care help shift the focus onto things that matter to our patients? Perhaps on the way we may need to make some compromises – human continuity for those who need it the most with informational approaches for others; greater access through technology and other routes but with fewer physical spaces and doctors; greater segmentation of our populations and resources and strategies targeted to their needs; and solutions for the organisation and delivery of healthcare that are created around the needs of patients and not healthcare providers.

Only the future will tell how we can overcome these challenges. But one thing is certain – without collaborating with patients and their communities, we will never realise the greater goal of 'complete physical, mental and social well-being and not merely the absence of disease or infirmity' (WHO, 1946).

REFERENCES

Allan, L.N. et al. (2018) The unfulfilled potential of primary care *British Medical Journal* 363(k4469): 192–194.

Appelby, C. and Deeming, J. (2001) Kings Fund https://www.kingsfund.org.uk/publications/articles/inverse-care-law (Accessed 15.5.19).

Bailey, J., Glendinning, C. and Gould, H. (2018) *Better buildings for better services: Innovative developments in primary care* National Primary care research and development centre, London: Taylor and Francis.

Billet, G. (2016) Apprenticeship as a mode of learning and model of education *Education+Training* https://doi.org/10.1108/ET-01-2016-0001.

Castle-Clarke, S. and Imison, C. (2016) *The digital patient: Transforming primary care?* Nuffield Trust November.

Chana, N. and Ahluwalia, S. (2014) Evaluating the care of patients with long term conditions *London Journal of Primary Care* 6(6).

Gunn, R. et al. (2015) Designing clinical space for the delivery of integrated behavioural health and primary care. *The Journal of the American Board of Family Medicine* 28(Supplement 1): S52–S62. DOI:10.3122/jabfm.2015.S1.150053.

Hallin, K., Henriksson, P., Dalén, N. and Kiessling, A. (2011) Effects of interprofessional education on patient perceived quality of care *Medical Teacher* 33(1): e22–e26. DOI:10.3109/0142159X.2011.530314.

Körner, M. (2016) Interprofessional teamwork and team interventions in chronic care: A systematic review *Journal of Interprofessional Care* 30(1): 15–29.

Machin, L.L. et al. (2018) Interprofessional education and practice guide: Designing ethics-orientated interprofessional education for health and social care students *Journal of Interprofessional Care*. DOI:10.1080/13561820.2018.1538113.

Mickan, S.M. and Rodger, S.A. (2005) Effective health care teams: A model of six characteristics developed from shared perceptions *Journal of Interprofessional Care* 19(4).

Pattison, S. and Pill, R. (2004) *Values in professional practice* Ch 14 (eds.), Abingdon, UK: Radcliffe.

Pettigrew, L.M., Kumpunen, S., Rosen, R., Posaner, R. and Mays, N. (2019) Lessons for large scale general practitioner provider organisations in England from other inter-organisational health care collaborations *Health Policy* 123: 51–61.

Roland, M. et al. (2015) *The future of primary care Creating teams for tomorrow: Report by the primary care workforce commission* Health Education England www.hee.nhs.uk/sites/default/files/documents/The%20Future%20of%20Primary%20Care%20report.pdf (Accessed 21.12.18).

Sorensen, M., Stenberg, U. and Garnweidner-Holme, L. (2018) A scoping review of facilitators of multi-professional collaboration in primary care *International Journal of Integrated Care* 18(3): 1–14.

Van Loenen, T. et al. (2016) Trends towards stronger primary care in 3 western European countries 2006–12 *BMC Family Practice* 17(59).

Watt, G. (2012) General practitioners at the deep end: The experience and views of general practitioners working in the most severely deprived areas of Scotland *Occasional Paper Royal College of General Practitioners*. April (89): i–viii, 1–40.

West, M. and Dawson, J. (2012) *Employee engagement and NHS performance* Kings Fund www.kingsfund.org.uk/sites/default/files/employee-engagement-nhs-performance-west-dawson-leadership-review2012-paper.pdf (Accessed 16.12.18).

West, M., Eckert, R., Passmore, B. and Steward, K. (2014) *Developing collective leadership for health care* Kings Fund www.kingsfund.org.uk/sites/default/files/field/field_publication_file/developing-collective-leadership-kingsfund-may14.pdf (Accessed 16.12.18).

Woodson, T.T. et al. (2018) Designing health information technology tools for behavioural health clinicians integrated within US based primary care teams *Journal of Innovation in Health Informatics* 25(3): 158–168.

Wong, P.S. et al. (2018) Assessment of attitudes for interprofessional team working and knowledge of health professions competencies for final year health professional students *The Asia Pacific Scholar* 3(1): 27–37 DOI: https://doi.org/10.29060/TAPS.2018-3-1/OA1064.

World Health Organization (1946) Constitution and principles www.who.int/about/mission/en/ (Accessed 23.12.18).